The Bird Flu Manual

To order additional copies, please contact us.
BookSurge, LLC
www.booksurge.com
1-866-308-6235
orders@booksurge.com

The Bird Flu Manual

Grattan Woodson, MD

2006

The Bird Flu Manual

TABLE OF CONTENTS

ACKNOWLEDGEMENTS

The author wishes to gratefully acknowledge the significant contribution made to this book by David Jodrey, PhD, who served as the pre-publication editor of my first book, *The Bird Flu Preparedness Planner.* Alison Janse, Executive Editor for HCI Books took that text and transformed it into the best selling book on the bird flu crisis in record time. For her hard work on that project, I will be eternally grateful.

Rhonda Mullen, PhD provided essential copy editing support for the Bird Flu Manual. Her skills led to many improvements in the style and accessibility of the book. Dianna Eden sight edited the book, which helped to make it easier to read, more internally consistent, and in conformance with the norms of English grammar. William Stewart, an engineer and private Alternative Energy Consultant helped me think through the practical consequences a family would face coping with a severe pandemic, some of which are presented in part III of the Bird Flu Manual.

Thanks to all of you who have used this work to help your family and friends prepare for what was once the unthinkable, the return of a severe influenza pandemic. Your kind words, and most of all, use of my work to help prepare for the pandemic has given me the enthusiasm to write more in-depth about this topic in the present book and for the www.BirdFluManual.com website. The comments and feedback provided by these readers has been an inspiration and important source of motivation for me to pursue this latest project. Writing a book can be a difficult and thankless task but not for readers like these.

Best regards,

Grattan Woodson, MD, FACP
June 16, 2006

This book is dedicated to those who wish to do what they can to prepare for the coming influenza pandemic.

PREFACE

The H5NI avian influenza virus is spreading across the globe on the wings of migratory waterfowl. Hundreds of millions of birds have died so far, either directly from this influenza strain or from the culling of infected flocks. Many more will succumb before this virus runs its course. It is in the nature of successful avian influenza strains like H5NI to follow a well-worn trans-species journey from the avian to the mammalian. Over countless millennia this virus' progenitors have made this ancient journey. H5NI, or bird flu, is only the most recent member to attempt the jump from birds to man. The virus has begun its gradual but not yet epidemic spread within the human population, turning up in one new country after another. As this manuscript is being written, human cases are occurring sporadically. Should the number of human cases accelerate, this increase would indicate that the disease has entered the final developmental stage leading to a human influenza pandemic. Bird flu is progressing rapidly toward this status. The changing behavior of bird flu and the new genetic material it is acquiring through mutation and recombination with other viral strains, point to an eventual pandemic influenza strain.

Most of my work as a practicing physician is spent managing patients' imprecisely known health risks. The common challenge is a patient who has a specific condition known to cause a disease that places them at risk for a severe consequence. Defining the risk as clearly as possible and then working on ways to lessen its effect on the patient is how I spend much of my time each day. In general, this approach is the one I've applied to the bird flu problem for this manual. Specifically, good evidence exists that another influenza pandemic has been brewing in Asia since at least 1997. However, it is unknown if the resulting virus will cause a mild, moderate, or severe pandemic. Neither can anyone predict accurately when such a pandemic will occur. Given the inevitable risk to health implied by a pandemic, prudence dictates taking reasonable steps to cope with the foreseeable consequences. Studying the history of influenza and the H5N1 viral strain led me to the conclusion that the bird flu virus is just one step away from attaining pandemic status and that this evolution could occur at any time. This development has the potential to be a grave threat to the health and safety of humankind, for which few people are prepared. Helping people come to terms with the risk we face from a pandemic and the steps necessary to cope with an emergency on this scale was my motivation for writing this book.

Part I of the manual provides background information on influenza with a tight focus on the H5N1 bird flu virus. This section presents a review of the evidence that the H5N1 virus is rapidly adapting to humans, supporting the concern that it could soon become pandemic. If a pandemic happens, it will affect people everywhere with consequences ranging from mild to catastrophic.

Part II of the manual provides you with a detailed discussion of the symptoms and signs of bird flu. It will teach you how to tell the difference between bird flu and other similar illnesses. This discussion is followed by specific recommendations for the treatment of these symptoms. The Department of

Health and Human Services in their Pandemic Influenza Plan states that a moderate or severe influenza pandemic will infect 90 million Americans. Part II of the manual addresses how to care for a sick adult or child with flu at home using a simple approach not requiring medical training. If the flu strikes, having this type of information at hand will be very useful. There is nothing exotic about this care. Most of the treatments presented rely on common sense, and most people will find the advice and suggestions similar to their own experiences. I explain exactly when, how, and why to provide various treatments, including use of over-the-counter medicines and a few select prescription drugs. *The Flu Treatment Kit* includes a list of items that will be of particular value in providing good home care to patients with flu, and most of the items on the list except for a handful of prescription drugs are widely available in grocery, drug, or even hardware stores.

The psychological health of many people will be severely threatened during and after the pandemic. No one will escape the touch of the pandemic. The manual includes suggestions for coping with these issues that do not rely on the availability of professional help or medications. It also includes ideas on how you can help your family remain sane in the face of an emergency of this magnitude.

More than anything else, the Great Bird Flu Pandemic will be a struggle for human survival. Part III of the manual is devoted to helping you make practical preparations to survive the pandemic. The lives of your loved ones and closest friends could well depend on how well you prepare. As demonstrated by the recent ineffectiveness of the federal government in coping with Hurricane Katrina, an effective government response to an emergency of this scope is unlikely. To depend upon public sources of aid and support during the pandemic would be unwise. Your family's survival will be best served by taking a self-reliant approach that includes making your own advanced preparations to cope with the illness and its predictable societal consequences. Given the stakes, the most prudent course of action is to prepare for the worst and hope for the best.

Preparing to handle the medical and practical consequences of a severe pandemic turns out to be more complicated than I expected. Going about the process in a haphazard manner could result in the exclusion of some critical items and the inclusion of others that are both frivolous and expensive. A logical first step is to draft a Pandemic Survival Plan for your family. This exercise will provide a rational structure to your preparation activities, and when done properly, it will help you get the supplies you really need at the best price and in a timely manner. Using a master plan makes sense and is my recommendation.

This emergency will be too big to face by individual families in isolation. What makes a lot of sense is for families, their friends, and neighbors to come together into a larger mutually supportive and sustaining Pandemic Support Group. Most people will be riding out the pandemic at home in their neighborhood, apartment building, or city block. Forming a group from among those living near you for the purpose of helping each other cope with this emergency is one of the best ways people can assure the survival of their family and friends. Even if one or both of the adults in a family are incapacitated, they can rely on other members of the group to take good care of their children as long as necessary. Throughout history people have responded to a crisis of this proportion in just this way.

The remainder of part III of the manual focuses on several practical concerns, with which you need to properly prepare your family to survive well during the crisis. For instance, an adequate supply of food and water during the pandemic will be necessary in the event of a breakdown of the usual sources of these items. What about lighting, cooking, and heating your home? How are you going to manage these problems if our conventional solutions fail? Part III of the manual tackles these issues. While not an exhaustive treatment, it provides an introduction to the topic that will at least get you on the right track. If nothing else, this section will help galvanize you to begin thinking about these issues and how you are going to solve them for your family.

An important point to keep in mind

The influenza pandemic is a real concern, and the more you study and come to terms with it, the more you understand this realization to be true. Commonly, people who make this journey experience some corresponding difficult psychological states. These stages usually unfold in a predictable manner, beginning with denial, fear, and anger, and then followed by grief and depression. This psychological transition is probably familiar to many of you who have gone through traumatic times. If you are already going through this transition or have yet to make this passage, the good news is that it does come to an end. A benefit of making this journey is that it can empower you to face this crisis with a calm determination that will provide you with an advantage during the emergency. As you inform yourself about the risks and take steps to improve your ability to cope with the practical challenges, you also are preparing yourself psychologically. Regarding the emotional strain all of us will experience as a result of the pandemic, a crucially important point is that *there is every reason to think that you and your loved ones will make it through this.*

The Great Bird Flu Pandemic, the name that will probably stick to this event, will surely be the seminal feature of the first half of the 21st century. We are all about to become the principal players in this drama of truly epic proportions.

The <u>WWW.BirdFluManual.com</u> website

This is a fast moving story with new developments every day. To manage this, I have sponsored a website to provide updates for the manual, where new information about the pandemic will be published on a regular basis. One of the most important items I plan to place on the website will be my assessment of the current Pandemic Alert Phase; a measure useful for triggering elements of your pandemic preparedness plan. These triggers are driven by changes in the H5N1 bird flu's behavior or developmental milestones, which is what I think is the best guide to current pandemic risk.

I have authored a variety of <u>Original Articles</u> for the Bird Flu Manual website. The topics covered by the original articles are all related to the pandemic and include some items discussed in the book but in greater detail. Underlined hyperlinks to the website are scattered throughout the PDF version of the book when there is an original article, resource, or item of interest that relates to a topic discussed in the book. To access these hyperlinks, make sure your computer is connected to the Internet then just double click on the link in the PDF and you will be taken to the proper section of website.

The Bird Flu Manual website has a <u>Feedback Section</u> where you can share your views, ideas, comments, and questions for me on the pandemic or the manual. These comments will be kept private, as I am not interested in hosting another bird flu forum—a service already provided superbly by others like www. fluwikie.com.

Having gone through the process of preparing my family and helping others get ready for the possibility of a flu pandemic, I have learned many lessons. Some are practical in nature such as what supplies to get and where to get them. Another section of the website is dedicated to this topic. In the Pandemic Preparedness Store, you will find a variety of items that may help you prepare for the pandemic. There are underlined context specific links to locations within the Pandemic Preparedness Store found in the PDF version on this book. While reading the PDF, if you click on one of these links it will take you to a section of the Bird Flu Manual website store containing one or more items related to the issues discussed in the text. The items displayed in the store are linked directly to the Internet address of the venders who sell them. To buy something seen in the store or find out more about it from the vendor is simple. All you need to do is click the item's link on the Bird Flu Manual website and you will be taken directly to that item's location upon the vendor's website. The store was developed to provide you with an idea of some of the solutions that are available for the potential problems we face from a severe pandemic. It also was set up to make it easier for you to shop by putting some the items you may need all in one place.

In the Resources Section of the website, I have placed a number of articles, pamphlets, booklets, and books in PDF format that are in one way or another related to the influenza pandemic. This collection of resources includes many of those I used during my studies and preparation for the pandemic and as source materials for writing on this issue. Many of the endnote references are stored in this section of the website. They cover a broad range of topics. In the PDF version of this book, there are links embedded at points in the text that will link you directly to a sections of the Bird Flu Manual Resource area that relates to that topic. This will allow you to quickly explore in more depth an area that you have a question about that is presented superficially in this book. For more information, an annotated guide to the Bird Flu Manual website is found in at the end of this book.

CHAPTER I

Part I: The Great Bird Flu Pandemic

A pandemic is simply a worldwide epidemic. During flu pandemics, a higher-than-usual percentage of the population becomes infected and more people die from these infections than during the annual flu season. Wild birds are the natural reservoir of the influenza virus family, and there are literally hundreds of different strains. Pandemics occur when one of the influenza virus strains makes its way from birds to humans, sometimes with an intermediate step in another mammal. Adaptation to humankind is a trial-and-error process for the influenza virus, which depends on natural selection and therefore takes time. It is common for influenza strains to cross over from the avian world to the mammalian. Most of the time nothing comes of this activity because the virus is unable to adapt sufficiently and spread itself within the new host species. About every 30 years one strain does succeed, causing a human pandemic. This successful transformation happens because the virus is completely new to our immune system, leaving us vulnerable to its effects. The immune system is our best defense against influenza and with time, it will acquire the ability to defeat the new flu strain, giving us an advantage. Like a seesaw, power over human life and death swings back and forth between the influenza virus and our immune system. This ancient battle has gone on for thousands of years.

A highly virulent and deadly new influenza virus strain is once again emerging in Southeast Asia that is of great concern. This new flu has all the hallmarks of one that will succeed in becoming pandemic in humans. Scientists call this new virus Type A H5N1 avian influenza virus, popularly known as bird flu. In the opinion of many experts, including Lee Jong-wook, MD, the late Director-General of the World Health Organization (WHO), H5N1 will successfully adapt to humans.[1] However, reasons for uncertainty remain. Until recently we have lacked the scientific tools to track this natural event. It is well known that several avian influenza strains have emerged over the past decade that did not become human pandemics. The truth is that no one knows for certain if the next pandemic will be caused by the current H5N1 bird flu strain or something else. In this manual I take the view that H5N1 will cause the next pandemic, an assumption for which there is a growing body of supporting scientific evidence. [2,3]

The best scientific study on the origins of the H5N1 bird flu strain indicates it first emerged in birds in Guangdong, China in 1996.[2,4] The world became aware of the potential threat of an avian influenza pandemic in 1997 when the disease first surfaced as "chicken flu" in Hong Kong. At the time 18 people became ill and 6 died, an unheard of occurrence with flu in recent times. The Hong Kong medical authorities traced the potent flu to diseased poultry. They slaughtered more than a million birds, and the virus disappeared. This intervention seemed to have nipped the disease in the bud until 2003, when it reappeared in Southeast Asia in three tourists who became ill after visiting China. Two died and H5N1 bird flu was found to be the cause of the deaths.[5,6] Since then the number of human cases and geographic spread of the virus has been gradually increased.

The more I learned about H5NI, the more concerned I became. Soon I began to understand why the infectious disease and public health community have always been so interested and at the same time worried about the potential for a new influenza pandemic.[7]

The history of influenza pandemics

Surprisingly, pandemics occur quite often—in fact, around three per century. Since 1590, there have been 10 confirmed and three suspected flu pandemics.[8] Every 100 years or so, a major pandemic occurs that is so severe it dwarfs everything else by comparison. By everything else, *I mean everything* including all other diseases, war, and starvation. The last major pandemic event was the HINI Spanish flu in 1918. During that pandemic more people died within 18 months than in all the past wars in human history! An event with an unpredictable periodicity is referred to as being *regularly irregular*. History is full of reports of events that could have been influenza pandemics. The first recorded description of a health event consistent with influenza pandemic comes from Greece in 412 BCE.[9] In 1157-1158, writers describe an infectious disease pandemic with symptoms consistent with pandemic flu. Despite reports from the 13th through the 15th centuries suggestive of influenza pandemics before 1590, the information available is too sketchy to draw reliable conclusions.

The regularly irregular history of influenza pandemics throughout recoded history lies behind what today's influenza experts say: "When it comes to the next pandemic, it is not a matter of if but instead a matter of when, which virus, and how bad will it be". At this point in our ignorance of influenza biology, no one is able to accurately give the answers to these key questions. Our fate is to sit with these uncertainties and the inherent risk, waiting for the next pandemic to begin.[10]

Influenza must complete its genetic adaptation to humans before it can become pandemic. The last step in this process is gaining the ability to spread easily from one person to another. Virologists refer to this as *efficient human-to-human transmission*. When this flu behavior is confirmed and there is sustained spread of the virus in multiple geographic world regions at the same time, the pandemic officially begins. So, among those in the know, there is no doubt that this or some other new avian flu virus will adapt to humankind and cause another pandemic. The burning questions are: will it be H5NI bird flu or some other flu strain, when will this happen, and how bad will it be?

The WHO Pandemic Influenza Alert Phases

The WHO has developed a warning system designed to alert the public about what is happening in the avian flu world.[11] The purpose of the system is to give the world a heads-up if a new strain is making its way down its evolutionary path to visit us again. National public health agencies also rely upon these phases to trigger individual plans. This alert system is a new and revolutionary idea. We never have had a warning system such as this in place, so we are about to see how well it works. As of June 2006, based on the bird flu cases officially recognized by the WHO, the alert phase is at 3 on a pandemic alert scale of 1 to 6. As the pandemic alert phase number rises, so does the risk of a pandemic. The WHO will declare Phase 6, the start of pandemic influenza, when they establish that efficient human-to-human transmission of the virus is occurring in several geographic regions of the world simultaneously. <u>Official Pandemic Plans</u>

WHO Pandemic Influenza Alert Phases

Inter Pandemic Period

- Phase 1. No new influenza virus sub-types detected in humans although there are some endemic in animals that have infected humans.
- Phase 2. No new influenza virus sub-types detected in humans, but a circulating animal subtype poses a substantial risk to human health

Pandemic Alert Period

- Phase 3. Human infections with a new sub-type, but no or only minimal human-to-human spread to close contacts.
- Phase 4. Small clusters with limited human-to-human transmission but spread is highly localized, suggesting that the virus is not well adapted to humans.
- Phase 5. Larger clusters but human-to-human spread still localized, suggesting that the virus is becoming increasingly better adapted to humans, but may not yet be fully transmissible (substantial pandemic risk).

Pandemic Period

- Phase 6. Pandemic: increased and sustained transmission in general population.

What WHO Influenza Pandemic Alert Phase are we really in?

Good evidence exists that some limited person-to-person spread has occurred regularly since the virus reemerged.[12,13,14] Since May 2005, scientists have reported small human-to-human clusters in China, Indonesia, Turkey, and Iraq. Progressive adaptation of the virus to humans may be responsible for its ability to pass more easily from birds to people, and in a limited way from person-to-person. Despite these developments, the WHO has kept the official alert status firmly on Phase 3. Further on in the text is a more detailed discussion of the reasons why the WHO Altert Phase should have been advanced to 4 in 2005.

The transition time between phases is something we cannot now predict. We don't understand what is happening because we are witnessing it for the first time. Nevertheless, I am concerned that as H5NI bird flu accumulates the genetic sequences it needs for pandemic status, its progression may accelerate toward the end of its evolutionary journey. The rationale for this thinking relates to the fact that the virus is spending more and more time reproducing in human and swine cells. The more time spent in these mammalian host environments, the more opportunity there is for the virus to obtain the missing hemagglutinin receptor for the human upper respiratory tract it needs to become pandemic. This can happen when bird flu and another strain co-infect the same host. Under these conditions, the H5NI could obtain this missing protein from another flu strain already adapted to humankind by means of exchanging genetic material with it.

H5NI is involved in an evolutionary process that favors the survival of the fittest viral strain. Natural selection is exerting pressure on the H5NI virus, favoring strains that reproduce well in humans. The odds of bird flu acquiring the missing receptor increase as the number of human infections rise. Since by definition, the number of human cases of influenza rises as the WHO pandemic phase increases, it seems logical to postulate that the pace of the virus's evolution will quicken toward the end of this process. In effect, if this view proves to be correct it means the time it takes for the virus to move through the final phases of its development will shorten. In practical terms this means that the time it spends in phase 5 will be less than phase 4. So, if we are already in phase 4 as I think likely, phase 5 may not be too far around the corner.

Like it or not, many governments have tied their national preparedness activities to the WHO Pandemic Alert Phase. This means that the time the world has to prepare for a bird flu pandemic is closely related to the WHO Phase. To the extent that this international body fails to advance the phase in a timely manner, all those who depend upon it for guidance are placed at increased risk. If it turns out that viral progress toward pandemic status accelerates near in the final stages of its journey, the time remaining for the world to prepare for a pandemic may not be as long as thought. The WHO, a creature of the United Nations, is under great pressure from many quarters regarding this issue and many others related to the pandemic. To the extent that these pressures are politically or economically motivated, they strike me as quite dangerous and terribly misguided. In my view, the WHO should be left alone to "call it like they see it" rather than having to hedge their opinions to accommodate interests unrelated to world health.

CHAPTER 2

Influenza Virology 101
Endemics, epidemics, and pandemics

A disease is *endemic* when it remains stable within a host population. In other words, it infects a fairly constant percentage of the population year in and year out. An example of an endemic disease in the United States is mononucleosis. Occasionally, a spike in the number of cases of an endemic disorder results in a small and usually self-limited epidemic. By contrast, an *epidemic* is an infectious illness that spreads so quickly that the number of new cases rises in an exponential manner rather than increasing linearly. During epidemics, the number of new cases doesn't just go up by one or two each day but rather doubles every few days.

A *pandemic* is an epidemic that spreads across the globe affecting people on every continent and is not confined to one geographic area. An ongoing H5N1 epizootic (a pandemic in a non-human animal species) has been occurring in the avian world since 2003 or before, with it now affecting birds across approximately half of the world. The persistently high mortality rate among birds infected with the disease is a disturbing phenomenon accompanying this epizootic.[5] Virologists regard this development as unprecedented. Typically, during the epizootic

9

phase of the infection, the mortality rate of the targets of the disease is much lower.

Cases of the disease are persisting in birds and mammals, including people, despite the best efforts of agricultural and public health officials to contain it. For students of influenza, this moment is an instructive one. Never before in human history have we been witness to the onset of an event so momentous as the development of a possible influenza pandemic. Since we've never experienced this event in this way before, it is unknown what the virus is doing or why. In the future, we will look back on this watershed endemic period and be able to recognize the role it played in the evolution of H5N1, which I believe is on the road to becoming a newly emergent pandemic influenza.

Pandemics vary in severity

There are mild, moderate, and severe influenza pandemics. During the 20th century, we have had one of each type.[15] All pandemics infect many times more people than happens with seasonal flu, but during a severe or major pandemic, deaths soar into the tens of millions. Mild and moderate pandemics are still severe by comparison to a typical annual winter flu season. For instance, the 1957 Hong Kong Flu was a moderate pandemic that caused three times as many deaths than during seasonal flu. However, the mild 1968 Asian flu pandemic caused only a few more deaths than a normal flu season. Thirty-eight years has lapsed since the last flu pandemic, which suggests we may be due for another one soon. Influenza Virology

The clinical attack and case fatality rate

During a major pandemic like the 1918 Spanish Flu, five to 10 times as many people as usual became severely ill with flu, and many millions died from their infection. The percentage of the population that becomes ill with flu symptoms is known as the *clinical attack rate.* Studies of influenza antibody levels in people's after the 1957 pandemic have revealed that the percentage of patients with exposure to the virus was approximately twice as high as the reported clinical attack rate for the epidemic. In other words, for every person who gets sick with flu during a pandemic, there is another person who contracts the virus but has no or few symptoms of the illness.

The medical term for the percentage of those who become ill and later die is the *case fatality rate.* The case fatality rate for flu hovers around 0.2% to 0.35%, a fraction of one percent, during the usual winter flu season. During mild to moderate pandemics, this rate can increase 3 or 4 times, but during a severe pandemic, the case fatality rate increases by 10 to 50 times.

As the virus spreads from one person to another, it can infect the new person only if that person is *susceptible* or vulnerable to it. Susceptibility to influenza boils down to whether you have *immunity* to it. The only way that a person can become immune to a virus is from either having prior infection with it or having been vaccinated against it. Immunity is learned by and stored within several specially adapted blood cell types called T and B-lymphocytes.

With respect to influenza, virtually 100% of the human population is susceptible to a new strain. However, scientists remain puzzled about why fully half of susceptible patients who contract the flu have no or few symptoms. In the future, an explanation of this phenomenon may lead to very powerful medical tools.

One of the most important reasons for influenza's success as a human invader is its *infectivity*. The infectivity of an organism is determined by how easily it is transmitted from one person to another. Infecting agents that can cause illness after a small exposure are more contagious than ones that require a larger exposure. Infectivity increases when infection can be passed between people without direct contact.

The most common method of flu transmission is by breathing air contaminated with virus. The virus gets into the air when a person coughs or sneezes. Flu also is transmitted by direct contact with someone already ill with the disease. This contact includes shaking hands or even touching something that the sick person previously touched such as a faucet or door handle.

In Southeast Asia, physicians have found bird flu virus in the pulmonary, nasal, and oral secretions of patients as well as in blood and feces.[16] Under the right conditions, flu can remain infectious for one to three days outside of the human body on surfaces such as counter tops or doorknobs.[17] In cold water, the virus can survive for up to a month.[18] Transfer of the virus can occur when a susceptible person touches a contaminated surface. Once on the hand, the virus usually enters the body through the oral route. This method of transmission underscores why hand washing is such an important infection control method.

Pandemic influenza occurs in waves

A feature of influenza pandemics that is under appreciated is their reoccurrence in waves.[15] During the waves, an exponential rise in the number of cases of flu occurs compared to relatively calm periods between waves. Like an ocean wave, the number of new influenza cases rises quickly, reaches a peak, and then rapidly declines. The 1918 Spanish flu (H1N1) was associated with three waves while the 1957 Asian flu (H2N2) and 1968 Hong Kong flu (H3N2) pandemics had two distinct waves each.

The reason for this wave behavior is unknown, but some scientists have attributed it to a change in the season of the year. Typically, a pandemic wave lasts two to three months. In past pandemics, the time between two waves was as short as three months to as long as nine months.

A point to keep in mind about pandemic waves is that they can vary greatly in intensity. During the 1918 pandemic, the deadly second wave, which lasted just 8 weeks, was responsible for more than 90% of the deaths for the entire pandemic. Predictions for the coming pandemic are made more difficult in light of modern medical interventions including advanced hospital care, respiratory ventilation, antibiotics, vaccines, and antiviral treatments. While we can be certain that the advance of scientific knowledge will make treatments more effective now than in 1918, it is also true that the manufacturing capacity for antibiotics, vaccines, and antivirals will certainly be unable to keep up with demand if the pandemic is severe. Deciding who gets these measures and who doesn't is going to be a difficult call.

While the flu season in the Northern Hemisphere predictably occurs from November through March, during pandemics, flu can vary from this script. The first wave of the Spanish flu began during this time and ended in March 1918. The killer second wave began six months later in September and ended in November 1918. The third wave began the next month in December and lasted until the spring of 1919.

Some researchers have speculated that one reason pandemics end is simply because all or most of the susceptible people within the population have contracted the infection and either died or developed immunity. Host species that have achieved this condition have *herd immunity*. The well-adapted pandemic influenza virus remains with its human hosts year after year from that time onward, becoming a new cause for seasonal flu—as evidenced by the three strains that became pandemic in the 20th century. Through the process of *antigenic drift*, these former pandemic strains change gradually, just enough to continue to cause seasonal flu. In time, a new pandemic strain crosses the species divide between the avian and mammalian world, becoming a new pandemic strain initially but then settling down to take its place as a new cause for seasonal flu.

Young adults suffer the most during pandemics

A major difference between seasonal and pandemic flu is the predilection pandemic flu has for healthy 15- to 40-year-olds. During the 1918 flu, society saw the highest death rates in this group with the peak between ages 20 and 30. By contrast, seasonal flu strikes hardest among the very old, the young, and those of any age with chronic medical conditions. Of course, neither are the usual victims of seasonal flu spared during pandemics. On the contrary, death rates are much higher for every age and risk group during pandemics compared with seasonal flu. The point here is that people between the ages of 15 to 40, who are usually immune to the ravages of seasonal flu, experience the highest case fatality rates of any group during severe pandemic years. Ironically, one possible explanation for this observation may relate to the increased health and vigor of the immune system of young people.

This idea is known as *cytokine storm* theory.[19] It holds that, in young adults, the immune system mounts a very intense response to influenza virus once it achieves the ability to respond to it. This response has taken several days, and in that time, the flu has reproduced many times within the patient's tissue, particularly in the lungs. The immune system quickly puts all its defenses into the fight against flu, including an array of specialized molecules used in immune defense called *cytokines* and several varieties of white blood cells. These mechanisms attack the free virus circulating in the blood and the virally infected lung cells directly.[20] While this immune response is making headway against the virus, it is doing so at a high cost to the remaining normal lung tissue that becomes, in a sense, the victim of "friendly fire".

As a result of this innocent bystander injury, the diseased and healthy lung tissue fills with fluid and becomes unable to absorb oxygen normally. The damage spreads quickly throughout the entire lung, resulting in a rapid death. The medical condition that develops is called Acute Respiratory Distress Syndrome (ARDS), which has other causes besides influenza and cytokine storm. ARDS is a disorder with which modern medicine has considerable experience but unfortunately unsuccessful results even under the best of circumstances. The case fatality rate for patients with ARDS from any cause treated in a U.S. hospital intensive care unit is about 50% today.

Cytokine storm is a *biologically plausible* but unproven explanation for the rapid deaths of so many young people during pandemics If scientists can establish it as the cause of ARDS during treatment of patients with influenza, they may be able to develop a way to prevent it. Currently, we don't know how to do this.

Pandemic flu spreads fast

Influenza is the king of pandemics. The infectious characteristics of influenza help explain why this organism can quickly spread from one region of the globe to another. Even during the relatively primitive travel conditions in 1918, it only took 6 weeks for epidemic influenza to spread from the United States to Europe and Africa. Imagine how fast the next pandemic virus will move across the globe given the many thousands of passengers traveling internationally by air every day. Facilitating this process will be the fact that infected people shed virus for several days before they have any detectable symptoms. Taking this silent phase into account, the British Government's Health Protection Agency predicts in their Influenza Pandemic Contingency Plan that once the first case of pandemic flu reaches Hong Kong, it will take only two to four weeks for the pandemic strain to arrive in the United Kingdom.[21]

The U.S. Department of Health and Human Services estimates that each person who contracts pandemic flu will pass it on to an additional two or three people.[22] It makes a big difference if the *transmission rate* is two or three because this number represents how fast the virus is passed from person to person. For instance, a viral spread with a transmission rate of three is passed from person to person exponentially faster than if the rate is two. The rule when dealing with pandemic flu is the more sick people you have, the more sick people you get. Any factor that increases the susceptibility of a population to the virus also will increase the transmission rate of the virus within the population. Official Pandemic Plans

In 1918, our world population was 1.6 billion and today it is 6.6 billion. Only 17% of the world's inhabitants lived in urban environments in 1918 and at the time there were only 15 cities with more than one million inhabitants. Today slightly less than half of humanity lives in urban settings that occupy only 3% of the earth's surface area and there are over 400 cities with a population of over one million.[23] *High population density* is a well-known and understood factor favoring epidemics, including influenza. The human species never has faced a major pandemic with such a large or geographically concentrated population. This factor alone makes predicting the magnitude of the impact of a major pandemic difficult. These population factors will worsen a pandemic, without a doubt, but by how much, we are unable to know.

Breakthroughs in agriculture, sanitation, nutrition, and medicine have combined to push the average life expectancy in the developed nations to about 80 years today from 50 years of age at the beginning of the 20th century. These advances have improved both quality of life as well as longevity. As a result, many people alive today would have perished had they been born in an earlier time. However, this magnificent achievement comes with an unintended consequence. To the extent that our populations have been enriched with medically frail members, its vulnerability to a pandemic virus increases.[24] The increase in risk affects both the healthy and the frail because the flu's transmission rate is enhanced in a population with a significant number of frail members.

It is becoming clear that wild birds are spreading the H5N1 virus across the globe along their traditional migration routes.[4,25] The best evidence suggests that about 2% of wild geese are the asymptomatic carrier or *vector* of a variety of strains for avian influenza, including H5NI bird flu. These waterfowl cover thousands of miles during their semiannual migration, spreading the virus as they go. In addition to being carried from wild birds to domestic poultry, the poultry trade itself also may be abetting the spread of H5NI infection. By the first quarter 2006, H5NI had spread throughout Asia and Eastern Europe and entered the Middle East, Africa, and Western Europe.[26] Soon it will reach North and South America and Australia in an expected pattern.

Most likely, we will see continued low-grade spread of the virus among animals and people in Eurasia, the Middle East, Africa, and North and South America. Nature has selected wild ducks as the primary carriers of this particular phase of the virus's pandemic genetic evolution. Once the virus achieves pandemic status, then the vector of the disease will move from birds to humankind. We will become the vectors of the pandemic strain of bird flu as we spread it person-to-person. Again, the spread pattern we are likely to see when human carriers become the vectors will follow well-known flyways, as was the case with the 2003 SARS outbreak. Only this time its passage will not be the wetlands and marsh of the wild duck but the jet ways and flight paths of the likes of Delta, British Airways, and JAL.

CHAPTER 3

Why is the H5NI Bird Flu so Fearsome?

What makes avian influenza H5NI so troubling to many is the stunning 50% case fatality rate reported for human cases of bird flu. The WHO and most national public heath authorities are keeping close track of these cases, their location, and the deaths due to bird flu. By the spring of 2006, more than 200 cases had met the WHO criteria for official recognition as a proven case, and among that group were approximately 100 deaths. Bird flu's terrifying 50% calculated case fatality rate is based solely upon these two numbers.

Bird flu lethality is overstated

The 1918 flu, like most pandemics, infected 30% to 50% of the world's population, or approximately 640 million persons at the time. If we assume that approximately 80 million people died during the 1918 influenza pandemic, we find a case fatality rate of approximately 12.5% of those infected.[27] While this estimate is terribly high, it is only a quarter of the 50% case fatality rate currently reported for bird flu. Medical References

Growing evidence indicates that the number of cases of human bird flu infections has actually been much higher, especially in the number of infections that were not fatal.[28] The undercount is partially attributed to conservative methods used by the WHO to confirm bird flu that predictably result in numerous false negative results and the lack of testing of less severely-ill cases of patients with bird flu.[29] Public health watchdogs in Vietnam, Thailand, China, Indonesia, Africa, the Middle East, and India have missed cases of bird flu since only those admitted to a hospital are tested routinely. In Turkey, WHO has stated that it intends to do a more thorough investigation of the outbreak, but as of the summer of 2006, it has not made findings public.[30] While bird flu may not be as deadly as once believed, that does not mean that we have nothing about which to worry. The U.S. government expects our way of life could be severely disrupted by a 2% case fatality rate, a conservative estimate. The consequences of a pandemic become exponentially greater as the case fatality rate increases.

When the bird flu re-emerged in 2003 as a human infection, it was localized in Vietnam, Thailand and probably Southeast China.[31] In Vietnam and Thailand, it infected a couple of dozen people, leading to 12 deaths, and in every case, those with the flu had close contact with infected poultry.

In 2004 the confirmed infection rate accelerated to about 100 cases, with 50 deaths in Vietnam, Thailand, and Cambodia. We have no information on human cases during that time in China although subsequent unofficial reports detail previously unknown outbreaks were occurring simultaneously in poultry.[4,32] In all of the officially confirmed cases, there was close contact between the people infected with sick poultry. The one exception was a case in the summer of 2004 where the only contact the person had was with an infected family member. This case became the first documented person-to-person spread of H5NI bird flu.[13]

Between May 2005 and November 2005 in China alone, evidence provided by unofficial sources shows more than 1,000 human bird flu infections and 310 patient deaths.[33] The exact number of cases or deaths and how many were examples of bird-to-man or human-to-human transmission is unknown due to the difficulty in obtaining samples from the right place at the right time. Both national governmental and international public health communities also have shown surprising reluctance to share information.[34,35]

In late June 2005, the first of a number of human cases of H5N1 developed in Indonesia.[36] By the fall of 2005, the individual cases were attributed to casual transmission of the virus from infected birds to man. These initial cases were followed several days later by one or two additional cases among the friends and family of the initial bird flu patients. In many cases, the newly ill had little, if any, contact with infected birds. Related cases such as these are *clusters* and are consistent with limited human-to-human transmission of the bird flu virus. The limited spread between people means the virus is unable to get very far from the originally infected person. This passage is an example of *inefficient transmission* of the virus. Additional but less than perfect evidence exist to show limited human-to-human spread of bird flu in Vietnam, Thailand, and probably Cambodia in the form of clusters of the disease since 2003.[12]

There is also epidemiologic evidence of flu-like symptoms occurring in people living in Vietnam for a six-month period between 2003 and 2004 who had contact with sick poultry. This study's principal finding was significantly more mild to moderate cases of a flu-like illness in people who had prior contact with sick poultry compared to those with no contact.[37]

Extrapolating this data to the whole of Vietnam suggests that as many as 700 mild to moderate cases of bird flu during that period were unseen by medical authorities because people were not sick enough to warrant hospitalization. The policy followed throughout Asia has been to limit testing for the H5NI virus to those people ill enough to be hospitalized.

As detailed above, evidence suggests that bird flu fails to approach a 50% case fatality rate, a statistic that overstates the true lethality to an unknown extent. For instance, if we add the additional 700 Vietnam from 2004 cases and the unofficial reports on the human bird flu cases in China in 2005 to the WHO total, the case fatality rates drop into the low 20% range. A finding like this drop is exactly what we expect to see as the bird flu adapts itself to humans.

Evidence of bird flu's adaptation to humans

H5NI bird flu is adapting quickly to humans. In June 2005, for example, bird flu was passed from birds to people visiting the Jakarta Zoo without any direct contact. In Indonesia, Turkey, and Iraq, we have seen numerous examples of limited human-to-human spread of the virus among close contacts of people who first became ill with the flu, known as the *index cases.* Remarkably, in the December 2005 Turkey outbreak, the size of the clusters was much larger than seen initially in Indonesia 6 months earlier. These characteristics were not features of the sporadic cases of bird-to-human transmission seen in Vietnam, Cambodia, Thailand, and Laos between 2003 and early 2005. Since mid-2005, the virus has become entrenched in China, Indonesia, and the Middle East with new human cases and deaths reported each week from these areas.[38] The "endemic phase" of viral evolution is new as well.

We also have seen a widening geographic spread of the disease. Since the beginning of 2006, dozens of countries in the Middle East, Europe, Africa, and Asia have confirmed the presence of the virus, some with proven concurrent human infections. Finally, an accelerating yet still linear increase in the number of confirmed human cases and deaths from bird flu has continued to occur. When considered together, these developments support the notion that H5N1 is rapidly adapting to human hosts.

Natural selection favors viral offspring with qualities that adapt better to hosts, including birds, non-human mammals, and people. The viral genetic adaptation of bird flu to the human species is occurring simultaneously in every geographic location and species that the flu infects, and not just in people. When genetic change is spread across so vast a number of hosts and geographies, the chances of it's acquiring just the right combination of factors needed to become pandemic increase significantly.

Studies published in the spring of 2006 suggest that H5N1 has acquired all but one of the genetic tools required to produce a human pandemic.[39] The lacking characteristic is the ability for the virus to bind and invade the cells that line the human nose and throat.[40] The completion of this cycle will require the virus to obtain a receptor for this tissue. Unfortunately, many currently circulating flu strains, including all those causing seasonal influenza, already carry this genetic sequence within the gene coding for one of the proteins displayed on the surface of the virus, hemagglutinin. Since widespread influenza viral congress is ongoing, with H5N1's role in the pageant growing, it is highly likely that H5N1 will eventually obtain the missing receptor sequence from another strain through the process of viral re-combination or reassortment.

The present H5N1 virus host range includes the avian, swine, feline, canine, and human species.[41,42,43,44] If bird flu gains the genetic sequence enabling it to attach and invade cells effectively within the human upper respiratory system, the adaptation process will be at an end as far as we are concerned. A bird flu virus emerging from that last evolutionary step will possess the ability to pass easily from person to person through the air. That event will mark the beginning of the next human influenza pandemic.

Estimates of pandemic illness and death

When compiling statistics about the number of cases of illness and death that could occur during a pandemic, we fail to capture the uniqueness of each person and value of their lives. The purpose of a mathematical exercise is to more accurately calculate the consequences that might be expected under various conditions. By considering these numbers, we can grasp the larger implications of a pandemic on the nation or world. This knowledge then forms the basis for making recommendations on how to prepare for a pandemic. No one is "only" a number, but numbers do matter. How many patients will be seriously ill with pandemic influenza affects how many hospital beds will be needed. In a nutshell – in a severe, or even a moderate, pandemic, we will have many more patients than available hospital beds.

It is impossible to accurately predict how lethal bird flu will be if it becomes pandemic. In the opinion of Michael Os-terholm, PhD,[45] writing in the *New England Journal of Medicine*, the most likely scenario for a severe pandemic is for an event that approximates the death rate seen during 1918 Spanish Flu.[20] On the other hand, if the pandemic bird flu strain that emerges causes a mild or moderate pandemic, this occurrence would not represent a dire threat to humanity or even lead to a significant disruption in our way of life. <u>Worst Case Scenarios</u>

We can predict the pandemic's impact if we know the percentage of people that will come down with the flu, the number who will die from their infection, and the size of the population that will be affected. These statistics are known as the clinical attack rate (CAR), the case fatality rate (CFR), and population respectively. The number of deaths expected is simply the product of these three values (CAR x CFR x Population = *Number of Deaths*). The fatalities rise as any of the factors in the equation go up. It is as simple as that.

During the typical flu season the clinical attack rate is about 10% with the case fatality rate of approximately 0.275%.[7] During influenza pandemics, both statistics increase many times over, explaining why the number of deaths goes up so high during these events. The U.S. Government projects a clinical attack rate of 30% for the next flu pandemic, whether moderate or severe.[46]

US DHHS morbidity estimates for the US during the next pandemic		
Case Fatality Rate Estimate	Clinical Attack Rate Estimate	US Deaths Estimate
0.23% (Moderate)	30%	207,000
2.1% (Severe)	30%	1,903,000
US Population 2005 = 296,000,000		
Adapted from the U.S. DHHS Pandemic Influenza Plan, November 2005		

Realistic adjustments to the official death estimates

In my view, the U.S. Government's estimate for the clinical attack and case fatality rates for the next pandemic are optimistic. Our population is highly concentrated in cities today, and crowding is a well-understood epidemic accelerant. The average age of the population is higher now than in any prior pandemic. Older adults, especially those with chronic diseases, are more susceptible to influenza infection and more likely to die from the flu.[47] These factors were omitted from the U.S. Government's model, and yet all of these characteristics increase the vulnerability of our population to influenza. In my view, the presence of such factors will lead to a higher clinical attack of 40% than the 30% estimate by the U.S. Department of Health and Human Services.

Furthermore, their Pandemic Influenza Plan assumes that U.S. hospitals will remain open and functional during the 18-month pandemic period and be capable of providing standard care to an additional 10 million Americans.[48] If the hospitals receive a steady supply of critical inputs, allowing them to function, where will they find additional staffed hospital beds to accommodate the new influenza patients? The patient outcomes projected in the U.S. Government's plan depend upon each patient admitted to the hospital receiving standard hospital care. This level of care in turn depends upon the patient occupying a staffed hospital bed with full access to resources and supplies, an unlikely proposition.

Even if hospital admissions were distributed evenly throughout an 18-month pandemic period, the hospital system would have difficulty accommodating this many additional patients. During pandemics, however, cases usually occur in several discrete waves. To expect our very limited hospital surge capacity to be able to take care of the number of critically ill patients seen during or between pandemic waves lacks foundation. My estimate is that only about one in three of those needing hospital care will receive it. As a result, seriously ill influenza patients who are unable to obtain treatment in the hospital will not heal as well as those that receive the standard hospital care.

The next table applies these two assumptions to the U.S. Government's pandemic model. The specific changes include increasing the clinical attack rate to 40% from 30% and recognizing that U.S. hospital surge capacity is very limited making it unlikely more than 1 in 3 critically ill patients that need a staffed hospital bed will get one. These two adjustments increase in the number of U.S. deaths during a severe pandemic by five times the rate seen in the unadjusted model (from 1.9 to 9.9 million Americans). This increase corresponds to an increase in the overall U.S. case fatality rate from approximately 2% to 8% during an 18-month major bird flu pandemic.

Adjusted US DHHS Pandemic Influenza Plan for prognosis, clinical attack rate and treatment setting*				
Prognosis Type	Patient Number	Prognosis by Clinical Attack Rate	Case Fatality Rates	Deaths Expected
Type 1	4,144,000	3.50%	83.33%	3,453,333
Type 2	6,512,000	5.50%	38.33%	2,496,267
Type 3	107,744,000	91.00%	3.67%	3,950,613
Total	118,400,000	100%	8.39%	9,900,213
*Assumes 40% clinical attack rate and treatment setting: 1/3 Hospital Setting & 2/3 Home Setting				

For the worldwide death number, McKibbin and Sidorenko in their Lowy Global Economic Pandemic Study projected 142 million deaths for a severe pandemic.[49] Dr. David Nabarro, the United Nations coordinator for avian influenza, told the press in October 2005 that the death toll from a severe influenza pandemic could reach 150 million. Dr. Osterholm's range of 180 million to 360 million is based on the current best estimate of world deaths during the 1918 event of 60 to 100 million deaths. This estimate is adjusted for an increase in the world's population from 1.6 to 6.6 billion people.

Estimates of morbidity and mortality worldwide from pandemic influenza		
Case Fatality Rate Prediction	Clinical Attack Rate Estimate	Deaths Worldwide Estimate
7.36	30%	142,000,000 [a]
5.7%	40%	150,000,000 [b]
6.8%	40%	180,000,000 [g]
13.6%	40%	360,000,000 [g]
World Population 2005 = 6,600,000,000, [a] Lowy Global Economic Pandemic Study Ultra Scenario, [b] UN Worst Case Severe Pandemic Projection, [g] Osterholm severe pandemic projection		

CHAPTER 4

Pandemic Vaccine and Drug Issues

Vaccination

Vaccination is the most effective method of protecting against viral infections and influenza in particular. Overall, vaccination is considered 70% effective in prevention this infection. The seasonal flu vaccine is a *trivalent* product meaning it contains viral proteins from 3 stains of flu. The usual recipe calls for 2 strains of type A and 1 of type B flu. The current method of flu vaccine manufacture entails growing live virus in fertilized chicken eggs and then separating the viral particles from the egg. The particles from all 3 strains are inactivated by heat, blended, and then mixed with sterile water to produce a total concentration 45 mcg of killed viral particle proteins in each ½ cc of flu vaccine.

Purified killed influenza vaccine is proven to be safe and effective for producing protection against seasonal flu infection. After vaccination, the body's immune system recognizes these viral proteins as foreign invaders and mounts a vigorous campaign to destroy them. Vaccination leads to the formation of immune system B-cells that make antibodies against the virus and T-cells and macrophages that search out and destroy the virus directly. After encountering these foreign proteins once during the vaccination process, the immune system cells have a "memory" of them. They can respond more quickly and effectively when they meet them again in an actual infection.

These cells remain on alert in various locations such as the tonsils, lymph nodes, and spleen as well as circulating in the blood. They are on guard for any sign that influenza has invaded the body. When they encounter a strain of influenza to which they have been sensitized, they react. The first stage is the release of message cytokines into the blood that calls other cells and tells them to multiply rapidly. Antibodies are formed that bind the flu virus, and killer T-cells and macrophages engulf the virus and sequester it in small vesicles containing toxic chemicals. These cells quickly mount a usually successful defense against the flu.

One common misconception about flu vaccination is that it prevents infection with flu entirely. This is not so. Flu infection occurs even if you have been successfully vaccinated against that strain of flu. What happens when a vaccinated person develops the flu is that instead of experiencing a serious and in some cases life-threatening illness, the resulting infection is much milder and shorter in duration, resembling a cold. Sometimes a vaccinated person has no symptoms at all when they contract the flu.

Producers take approximately six months to make a batch of vaccine using the fertilized chicken egg method. In fact, the capacity to manufacture vaccines has been in decline here and abroad for two decades.[50] Today, world influenza vaccine capacity is just 300 million doses for seasonal flu, which is only enough to protect 5% of the human population.[7,15] Most of the world's influenza manufacturing capacity is in Europe (Great

Britain and France), the United States, Canada, and Japan. Two companies make seasonal flu vaccine in the United States, Sanofi Pasteur (with a capacity for 60 million doses) and MedImmune (that can manufacture about 3 million doses).

During a 2005 human vaccine trial with an experimental H5NI strain, Sanofi Pasteur made an unexpected discovery. For unexplained reasons the N5NI strain did not stimulate a very strong response from the human immune system. It took a vaccine dose that was six times greater than the seasonal flu dose of bird flu virus to obtain a protective immune response.[51] In addition, the dose had to be divided into two separate injections given 3 weeks apart to achieve immunity. Scientists are working on ways to increase the *antigenicity* or immune stimulating properties of the vaccine by combining it with another substance called an *adjuvant*.[52] Adjuvants are compounds mixed with antigens that provoke a more intense immune response from the antigen. In the meantime, Glaxo Smithkline discovered another complication. The industrial yield of H5NI viral particles grown in fertilized chicken eggs was reduced by 20% to 50% compared with the yield when growing seasonal influenza. Apparently bird flu is so lethal that it kills the chicken embryo in the egg before enough time has passed to raise a good yield of viral particles.

Today people living in the eight wealthiest countries consume 90% of the influenza vaccine manufactured worldwide. The looming bird flu pandemic has brought this inequity in vaccine manufacture and distribution into tight focus. A similar problem in the supply and distribution of antiviral drugs are disturbing to many people, especially those living in the less developed nations. This has led to the reluctance of some governments in Asia to share their viral samples with scientists in the

West unless it is understood that the West will share any vaccine derived from these specimens with the East.

No current bird flu H5N1 vaccine

No current H5N1 vaccine is specific for the future H5N1 bird flu pandemic virus.[7,10,11,20,22] Bird flu has not yet adapted enough to become pandemic, meaning that more genetic change is required before it achieves that status. Genetic changes in the virus are often reflected in the shape and composition of the proteins that cover the surface of the viral particle. Our immune systems are very specific. Antibodies formed against a specific invading viral strain are not very active against the same strain that has undergone even small changes or genetic drift as it mutates.

While vaccination is our best hope of avoiding catastrophe, we know that none will be available when the first wave of the pandemic spreads across the globe. In all likelihood, the first wave of such a pandemic will be characterized with a high rate of infection and many deaths. The time between the first and second wave is crucial. We need time for the manufacturers to brew enough vaccine to protect as many of the remaining susceptible population as possible.

Best case scenario for a bird flu vaccine

Most likely, pharmaceutical researchers will be able to increase the vaccine's antigenicity by 100%, possibly by combining it with an adjuvant. What's more, pharmaceutical companies can produce two batches each year with the first batch rolling out of the manufacturing plant 6 months after the isolation of the pandemic flu strain. Another important technical hurdle is the need to *attenuate* or weaken the flu virus in a way that will prevent it from killing the chicken eggs but not in a way that will reduce the viral protein's immunogenicity for the pandemic strain.[53] Making these assumptions then, the best-case vaccine production using the current egg-based technology is 300 million 45-mcg doses every 6 months beginning at the start of the pandemic.

To accomplish this level of production, we must make the following four assumptions:

- The manufacturers will have access to 300 million fertilized chicken eggs every six months for use in making the vaccine.
- The pandemic H5N1 strain is available for culture.
- The pandemic H5N1 strain can be made non-lethal (attenuated) to chicken eggs.
- The non-lethal H5N1 strain remains specifically immunogenic for pandemic H5N1 bird flu.
- The immunogenicity of H5N1 can be at least doubled by combining it with an adjuvant.

Assuming that these critical conditions can be realized in a timely and efficient manner, the worldwide vaccine production would equal 300 million effective courses every six months. The number of 300 million effective vaccine courses is based on the following:

- 22.5-mcg of viral antigen plus adjuvant is required for each flu shot (three times the seasonal flu shot dose).
- The dose must be given twice with a 21-interval between doses. (It takes more antigen and two doses to achieve immunity with H5N1.)

Since pandemic vaccine will be in extremely short supply around the world, probably all available supply manufactured in a country producing it will be nationalized for use solely within that country. Using these best-case assumptions, the United States, for instance, would have about 60 million effective courses of bird flu vaccine rolling off the manufacturing line every six months. During the 18-month estimated duration of the pandemic, the United States would be able to vaccinate 120 million Americans out of a population of 300 million.

Antiviral drugs for influenza

Roche Pharmaceuticals sells oseltamivir under the trade name of Tamiflu®.[54] Tamiflu works best if started within the first 48 hours of the beginning of the illness. The drug should be reserved for treatment of those who become ill with flu rather than being used for prevention to protect adequate supplies.

As reported in the journal *Nature* in May 2005 and the *New England Journal of Medicine* in February 2006, some strains of H5NI avian influenza infecting humans in Southeast Asia are developing resistance to Tamiflu.[55,56,57]

Tamiflu resistance occurs as a result of the virus undergoing a mutation in the neuraminidase gene. While making this change allows the flu to escape the effect of Tamiflu, it also partially cripples the virus by making it much harder to infect the cell and kill it.[58] In other words, bird flu without the Tamiflu resistance mutation is much more deadly than those flu viruses with it. So, Tamiflu could be useful for treatment even if there is a high prevalence of Tamiflu-resistant avian influenza strains in the community. The drug would select out the weaker members of the viral family as the ones that got through the Tamiflu defense while screening out the stronger members. Influenza Drugs

Probenecid is a medication approved by the U.S. FDA for treatment of gout and increasing the blood levels of penicillin-like drugs.[59] Many physicians use it off-label to increase the plasma level of drugs taken to treat malaria, meningitis, tuberculosis, and HIV/AIDS.[60,61] In test subjects given probenecid in combination with Tamiflu, the blood concentration doubled, and the time Tamiflu remained active in the body increased by a factor of 2.5, from eight to twenty hours.[62,58] In effect, if Tamiflu is given in combination with probenecid, you can get the same benefit using only half the dose otherwise needed. Medical References

Relenza is also a neuraminidase inhibitor and is probably effective against H5NI.[63] The drug is a powder and requires inhaling into the lung using a handheld device. Relenza is expensive, and manufacturing capacity for this product is quite limited. Most, but not all, strains of H5NI are resistant to the other older anti-influenza drugs like amantadine. So, other than a specific vaccine that has not yet been developed, and the antiviral drug Tamiflu and Relenza, no other effective treatments for H5NI exist. However, many important, lifesaving supportive therapies that I will share with you in the next chapters can mitigate your reaction to bird flu. In March 2006, the U.S. FDA approved the use of Relenza for treatment of H5NI.

Shots and boosters

Even though the recipe for the seasonal flu vaccine lacks protection against the H5NI flu, be sure to get one anyway. Many experts predict that the most likely time for the pandemic to begin is during the regular flu season. If you have the flu shot, it will protect you against the seasonal flu at the same time that pandemic flu may be circulating in your community. Also, no one wants to have flu twice in the same year.

✈ You can protect yourself from pneumococcal pneumonia by getting a Pneumovax vaccination. One of the many ways flu kills its victims is by setting the stage for them to contract pneumococcal pneumonia. Being vaccinated against this important cause of death and other common infections of children and adults will be important in the event that we experience a major flu pandemic. If you have already had one Pneumovax shot in the past, a second one is usually unnecessary.

All adults need a Tetanus/Diphtheria/Pertussis booster every ten years.[64] Pertussis is the organism that causes Whooping Cough and is the cause of chronic cough in both children and adults. While most adults receive vaccination for this disease as a child, the immunity gained only lasts 10 years, requiring a booster shot. Your doctor will be able to give you all these shots or advise you where you can get them.

Stock up on regular medications

We may experience shortages or the temporary unavailability of many key drugs during pandemic. This scenario is likely to coincide with the height of the pandemic when drug production and distribution could come to a temporary halt. Pharmaceutical manufacturing during the 18-month pandemic will experience production interruptions due to shortages of basic materials and absentee staff. Getting these complex facilities up and running again will take much longer than the time they were closed because of safety, regulatory, and legal concerns. Some medical conditions are simply so severe that they need to be treated continuously even during a bird flu emergency. Others while important to long-term health or present comfort may be ignored in the short term without too much harm. For critical medication, a prudent course is to stockpile a three- to six-month supply.

Those who are able to establish a stockpile would still purchase their regular 30- or 90-day supply of medications for day-to-day use. Rotate your drug stock so that each time you pick up a new prescription, put it in your stockpile and pull out a month's worth of the same drug with the least amount of time left before expiration. Almost every drug is still good after its expiration date; so don't concern yourself too much about expiration dates.

Medications in the critical "must take" category include those for chronic medical conditions like diabetes, hypertension, emphysema, chronic bronchitis, asthma, coronary artery disease, and hypothyroidism. There are many other conditions that treatment must be continued during the pandemic period. My advice is to contact your doctor and get a prescription for at least three-month's supply of the medications that fall into this category and have this stockpile on hand in addition to a regular supply. Discuss this with your doctor.

For critical medication you and your doctor think you must continue to take during the pandemic period, a prudent choice is to establish a three- to six-month stockpile of the medication now.

Women who are of childbearing age and sexually active should consider what to do about contraception during the pandemic. During past influenza pandemics, pregnant women had some of the highest mortality rates of any group. If you are currently using birth control pills, the supply of these drugs could be affected in the same way that others are. Stocking up on an alternative contraceptive method like condoms or a diaphragm is probably the most prudent and cost-effective course to take.

Patients with organ transplants, insulin dependent diabetes, rheumatoid arthritis, AIDS, systemic lupus erythematosis, other connective tissue diseases, and those taking anti-coagulants will represent special management considerations during a pandemic emergency. This issue should be discussed with your doctor who may be able to help find available options even during the emergency.

People on major tranquilizers for thought disorders such bipolar disorder and schizophrenia should get a six-month supply of medication. Similarly, patients on antidepressants for either depression or anxiety disorders will need to continue these medications during the crisis.

Chronic medical conditions for which medical therapy is optional--meaning that it may be possible to go without treatment in the short-term without much harm--include cholesterol lowering drugs, arthritis treatment, and medication for GERD (indigestion and heartburn), migraine headaches, sleeping pills, osteoporosis treatments, and hormones. Some patients on anti-seizure medications may find that they can cope without their medication. They may have a seizure but as long as they are not driving, they can survive. If a patient's seizures are frequent without treatment, the patient should obtain enough medication for six months.

The important advice about medications ultimately needs to come from your doctor. She or he is the only person who can competently guide you in these matters. My purpose in writing about pharmaceutical use is not so much to tell you what to do as to give you a heads-up that this issue could surface for you and you should be prepared.

CHAPTER 5

Part II: Home Treatment of Influenza

The U.S. Government predicts that eight out of nine patients sick with flu will be treated at home. Home care is independent of high technology equipment, trained staff, sophisticated supplies, or even a functional electric grid. No hospital can function with the loss of any of these critical inputs. The home care model is able to adapt rapidly to changing conditions and continue to operate, while the hospital model is more rigid and slower to adapt. The enormous capacity of a home-based treatment system can easily encompass the entire population of people expected to become ill with bird flu rather than the small percentage the hospital model can serve.

Under severe pandemic conditions, if our hospital system becomes overwhelmed, an alternative approach to providing healthcare to the critically ill will be needed. In my opinion, the U.S. hospital system has the capacity to accommodate no more than one third of the additional 10 million patients the U.S. Department of Health and Human Services predicts will need hospital care due to flu. While the outcomes of patients treated at home may fail to be as successful as patients treated in the hospital, for some people, home care may be their only option. It need not be the last resort of the desperate. On the contrary, home care can be a reasonably good alternative to conventional hospital care, especially if those providing it are given the information needed and have the simple supplies available to accomplish this task.

In the United States, there are about nine million health care workers who are, for the most part, dedicated to their mission of helping patients. Undoubtedly these professionals will remain at their posts as long as possible. At some point, however, it is likely that many hospitals, clinics, and offices will close. Therefore, a natural shift will occur, with these trained professionals helping their friends, family, and neighbors who become ill with flu and have no option other than home care. The formation of ad hoc neighborhood health networks by health professionals is one way to leverage various medical skills and resources for the benefit of the community. Clearly, medical professionals have invaluable training and experience to contribute during a pandemic.

Neighbors' coming together for the purpose of providing mutual support during an emergency happens all the time. The process is normal and natural and will occur spontaneously during a pandemic. But it can be more effective if a little planning is in place. Healthcare workers should consider taking an active role in helping their neighborhood prepare for the pandemic.

What is "good home care" for flu?

Good home care is nine parts common sense and one part simple medical practice, and it does not require any healthcare training or background to implement. Taking care of someone with flu will be a familiar task for those who have nursed family members back to health in the past. Of course, healthcare workers with direct patient care experience and training will be adept in setting up a viable neighborhood health network. They will immediately understand the principles and practices of good home care. Good home care of bird flu patients is not dependent on high-tech capacities. Rather, the care relies on simple common treatments and techniques.

Despite the best efforts of the ad hoc neighborhood health team, critically ill patients will be better in a staffed hospital bed. Yet *organized care given well at home will be significantly better than no care or haphazard care in a hospital.*

This part of the manual focuses on caring for people with flu at home. It also includes suggestions for experienced healthcare workers on how to use simple household or hardware store items to administer advanced treatment options for the critically ill at home. An effective neighborhood health network system will require some basic supplies and tools, and some prescription drugs should be a part of the preparation.

The Flu Treatment Kit

Providing good care to family members and friends sick with influenza is a task that will be easier with a good supply of select over-the-counter medications, some medical equipment, and a few items from the grocery or hardware store. These items form the basis of the Flu Treatment Kit (FTK). In addition, a handful of prescription medications, obtained with your doctor's assistance, will be of value in managing many of the symptoms and complications of severe influenza. Your doctor may have other suggestions, especially since he or she knows your specific medical condition. The quantities recommended in the FTK are more than adequate for most situations.

The Flu Treatment Kit items for one person

Grocery store items

- Table salt: 1 lb (for making ORS, gargle and nasal wash)
- Table sugar: 10 lbs (for making ORS)
- Baking soda: 6 oz (for making ORS and nasal wash)
- Household bleach, unscented 2 gal (for purifying water and cleaning contaminated items) *Bleach Gel.*
- Caffeine containing tea, bags or dry loose: 1 lb (for treatment of respiratory symptoms)
- Two 8 oz plastic baby bottles with rubber nipples[65] (for administering ORS to severely ill)
- Two 16 oz plastic squeeze bottles with swivel nozzles (for administering ORS to the ill)
- Two Kitchen measuring cups with 500 cc (two cup) capacity (for measuring lots of things)
- One set of kitchen measuring spoons 1/8 tsp up to 1 tbsp (for making oral solutions and dosing)
- Fifty Soda Straws (for administering fluids easier)
- One Composition-Style Notebook (for keeping a medical record on the patient)

. Hand Gel.

FTK Items found at the drug store

- Petroleum jelly 4oz[66] (for lubrication of tubes, suppositories, and skin treatment and protection)
- Cocoa butter, pure 2 oz[67] (for making suppositories and skin treatment and protection)
- An accurate bathroom scale (for weighing)
- Two Electronic thermometers[68] (to measure temperature)

- Automatic blood pressure monitor (to measure blood pressure)
- Humidifier (for increasing the relative humidity of the air breathed by the patient)
- Pill cutter (to make it easier to reduce the dose of medications if desired)
- ✓ 1 box of Latex gloves # 100, (to help reduce contamination and spread of the virus and bacteria)

Non-Prescription drugs

- Ibuprofen 200mg (Motrin®) # 100 tablets (for treatment of flu symptoms)
- Diphenhydramine (Benadryl®) 25mg capsules # 100 (for treatment of flu symptoms)
- Robitussin DM Cough Syrup® or its generic equivalent (12 oz) (for treatment of cough)
- Acetaminophen 500mg (Tylenol®) # 100 tablets (for treatment of flu symptoms)

Miscellaneous FTK items

- Teakettle[69] (for steam therapy)
- 1 pint 95 proof grain alcohol (ethanol for use in making cough syrup and oral medicated solutions)[70]

FTK Items found at the hardware store

- ✓ N-95 masks #20 (2boxes) (to reduce diseases spread to and from the patient)
- ✓ 50 gallon sturdy plastic garbage container with top (used to store clean water for drinking)

FTK prescription drugs

- ✓ Tamiflu 75mg # 20: (for treatment of Bird Flu)[71]
- Probenecid 500 mg #20: (used to increased the blood level and half-life of Tamiflu)
- Promethazine 25mg (Phenergan®) tablets # 60 (for nausea, vomiting, abdominal cramping, and nasal congestion)
- ✓ Hydrocodone 5 mg with acetaminophen 325 mg (Lortab-5®) # 60: (for pain and cough)
- Diazepam 5mg (Valium®) # 60: (for treatment of anxiety, muscle aches, and insomnia)
- Azithromycin 250 mg (Zithromax, Z-pack®) # 20: (for treatment of bacterial pneumonia, sinusitis, or ear infections complicating influenza)[72]

Abbreviations: lb = pound, oz = ounce, gal = gallon, # = number, cc = cubic centimeters, tsp = teaspoon, tbsp = tablespoon, mg = milligrams, hrs = hours

Within the medical community questions of safety and ethics arise around giving patients prescriptions for medications such as those recommended in the FTK for stockpiling for an event such as influenza pandemic.[57,73] The controversy includes a concern that if everyone obtained a stockpile, the drugs would be unavailable for current use by those who are actually sick. Another reason public health officers and physicians refrain from giving antibiotics (azithromycin) or antivirals (Tamiflu) to patients for future use is a fear that patients will misuse the drugs. Misuse includes: taking antibiotics designed for bacteria to treat a viral infection (a fruitless practice); taking an inadequate dose of the antibiotic by either taking it too few times each day or not taking it long enough; and splitting the prescription between two people so neither one gets any benefit. Some physicians are opposed to giving patients access to a limited supply of controlled substances for treatment of flu symptoms. Influenza Drugs, Medical References

In my opinion, the risk is low that people seriously focused on preparing for a potential influenza pandemic are likely to abuse the privilege of having a stockpile of a few drugs. On the contrary, there is every reason to believe that they will use these drugs wisely and appropriately. Using drugs properly requires that patients have clear guidelines for when to use them, how much to use, how often, and for how long. These instructions are included in this section of the book, but the physician writing the prescriptions has the final authority and responsibility to determine if, how, and when these drugs should be used. An escalating pandemic risk will cause more doctors to understand the wisdom of prescribing such medications for their patients to have on hand in preparation for an emergency. Medical References, Original Article.

In the meantime, obtain all the other items on the FTK. These non-prescription items form the real foundation of influenza treatment with the prescription drugs serving a supporting role.

Caregivers at home need to learn how to obtain vital signs, including pulse, blood pressure, temperature, weight, and respiratory rate. Blood pressure is easily measured using an automated blood pressure monitor. These devices come with instructions that clearly explain how to use them. The pulse is provided on the blood pressure monitor readout. It can be measured directly by feeling the pulse at the wrist and counting how many beats pass in 15 seconds and multiplying by 4. Temperature is measured directly with a digital thermometer. The patient's weight is measured on a scale in the standard manner and is best taken with the patient lightly dressed without shoes and around the same each time each day. Watching for and counting the breaths taken over a 15 second period and multiplying by 4 is how you measure the respiratory rate. "Practice makes perfect" applies to learning and perfecting these skills.

Prognostic types and use of triage

One difference between seasonal flu and a major pandemic is just how hard the pandemic flu hits patients and how rapidly it kills. Patients affected by the flu are broadly categorized into three prognostic types. In medicine, the term *prognosis* means the likely outcome for the patient with the disease. Prognostic Type 1 patients are at high risk of dying from influenza no matter where they are treated. Type 2 patients will do well in the hospital but poorly at home, and Type 3 patients will do well in the hospital and fairly well at home.[74] A thorough discussion of prognostic types can be found in an <u>original article on the BFM. com website</u>.

As a general rule everyone should receive the same level of supportive care no matter their prognostic type. This support includes fluid treatment, medications for pain relief and comfort, a clean warm bed, and as much caring and reassurance as you can spare. Following this course of action is rational because we can't predict who will survive, especially early in the course of the flu. If the hospital is open and you have a Type 1 or Type

2 patient on your hands, take them there as soon as possible. If critical medical supplies are in short supply, especially the antiviral drug Tamiflu or the antibiotic azithromycin, the decision on how to ration these resources is best made by health professionals if they are available. If not, use your best judgment.

When it comes to using scarce medical resources, if the doctor's office and hospitals are closed, you will be required to make care decisions on your own. It is necessary to make difficult choices because when done properly, more people will benefit. Do the best you can and get on with your duties.

How flu is passed person-to-person

Don't worry about contacting the flu because it will contact you. The entire human population will be *susceptible* or vulnerable to infection with this new pandemic virus because our immune system has no prior experience with it. The human species has had many visits from pandemic influenza through the millennia. While our immune system may be caught off guard initially, it will rapidly bounce back and come to our defense. Pandemic influenza is so infectious, it is quite natural for the majority of the population to contract the virus before it is brought under control by the immune system. About half the people who contract the virus will have typical symptoms, and the other half will have very few, if any, symptoms. So, while virtually 100% of us are susceptible to this new strain, for reasons that we do not understand at present, only approximately two in five people will become clinically ill with the flu, two in five will get the virus but will not get very sick from it, and one in five will escape the virus altogether.

Another reason seasonal and pandemic flu is passed so easily from person to person is that people infected with the virus are symptom-free for a day or two after they become contagious. Once symptoms begin, adults remain contagious for about five days, but children and those with impaired immune systems often remain contagious for up to two weeks. We really don't know if or for how long people who show only a few symptoms are contagious.

The most common way for flu to be transmitted is by breathing air contaminated with virus. Coughing or sneezing is how the virus first enters the air. The closer people are to one another, the easier it is for the virus to spread, thereby making crowding a pandemic risk factor. Flu also can be transmitted by direct contact with someone ill with the disease through touching the person or something they touched. Once on your hand, the virus usually gains access to the body by mouth, entering the body through the gut. Flu can be transmitted if an airborne droplet containing viable virus lands in your eye where it gains access to tiny vessels on the surface of the globe or underside of the lid. The same is true if a droplet containing the virus lands in your open mouth. Under warm and humid conditions, the influenza virus can remain infectious on surfaces like counter tops or doorknobs for a couple of days.

One of the unique features of human cases of bird flu reported from Asia is that it causes diarrhea more often than seasonal flu. This presentation will probably become less important once H5NI develops the ability to attach itself to the upper respiratory tract. When entering the body through the gut, the virus reproduces in the intestine and releases millions of copies of itself into the loose stool of the patient, causing a very contagious bloody diarrhea.

If you can avoid being around anyone with clinical influenza, you may delay getting ill. However, if you are needed to provide care for a sick family member or friend with the virus, this strategy is impossible. The avoidance strategy also will leave you unprotected from those who are contagious but have yet to show any symptoms of the disease. Even if you were able to reverse quarantine your family in a secure, well-provisioned location until the pandemic waves had all passed, when you re-entered civilization, you would quickly become ill with pandemic influenza. This happens because the influenza virus remains with its new host population until it simply becomes too weak to cause infections. Then it is replaced by a new strain. If a vaccine were available, perhaps your sequestered family could receive it before re-entering society. While this strategy might work, it would be difficult to implement practically. Ultimately, most people are likely to be exposed to the virus. It's just a matter of time.

Wearing latex gloves and an N-95 mask when caring for the ill and changing your clothes, mask, gloves, and shoes when you leave a sick person's area is a way to protect parts of the house where healthy people live. In truth, pandemic influenza is so infectious anyone taking care of sick folks in their homes will be exposed repeatedly to the virus no matter what measures taken. As needed care is provided to family, friends, and even sick strangers, the caregiver will be exposed to infectious viral particles when assisting patients in the bathroom, changing bed linen, and washing soiled clothes. Simply breathing the air in the vicinity of the sick will result in significant exposure. Since most people will have one or more sick family members or friends to care for, it is unlikely to avoid exposure. Exposure during a pandemic simply can't be helped. Home Preparedness

The U.S. DHHS Pandemic Influenza Plan recommends use of a protective facemask to prevent the exposure to the caregiver as well as exposure to the patient and from pneumonia-causing bacteria some people carry asymptomatically within their respiratory tract. The N-95 mask is similar in appearance but very different in function to the simple surgical cone mask. The N-95 mask is designed for biological protection. It is one of the best ways to avoid inhaling the virus. You can buy these on the Internet and in hardware stores in the painting section. While the CDC infection control guidelines recommend that the masks be used once and then discarded, under the shortage conditions expected during the pandemic, this advice requires rethinking. The mask can probably be worn for several days before recycling since it is being used for flu prevention.

Two common surgical facemasks are available in the United States. The newer cone-type surgical mask and a flimsy rectangular mask are both designed to prevent the wearer from coughing on the patient during surgery and passing on an infection. Because they do not filter the air you breathe, it is not particularly useful as a way to prevent the wearer exposure to flu. Only the N-95 mask provides reliable protection from inhaling the influenza virus.

During the 1918 pandemic, rectangular surgical masks were thought to be an effective means of preventing spread of bacterial pneumonia as secondary infections in patients with lungs already weakened by flu, but this theory was never proven scientifically.

While not recommended by the manufacturer or the FDA, facemasks can be purified and reused during the pandemic. These simple medical devices are already predicted to be one of the first items to become scarce during a pandemic emergency. To recycle the mask, simply dip it in a 1:100 bleach solution and allow it to air-dry. The bleach will destroy paper and cloth masks eventually, but you should be able to get several uses out of them before this happens. You also can place the mask in a microwave oven on high for a minute. This treatment is likely to destroy all living organisms that have adhered themselves to the mask. Another approach is to place the mask in a solar oven long enough to dehydrate and heat-kill the virus and bacteria that contaminate it.

Coughing and hand washing etiquette

The U.S. Government recommends two simple but effective suggestions for reducing spread of the virus. These include covering your nose and mouth with a tissue or handkerchief when coughing or blowing your nose and by washing your hands after you have any contact with a sick person. Coughing or sneezing into your hands is not recommended because then you are liable to spread the virus to anything you touch with them. Instead, if a handkerchief is unavailable, cough or sneeze into the inside of your elbow or the sleeve of your upper arm.

Studies now show that the best way to wash your hands after coming into contact with an infected patient is to use the new waterless gel alcohol antiseptics. The gel is especially convenient when going from patient to patient or from the sick room to non-infected areas of the house. These gels are sold widely in drug stores, but while inexpensive, they do cost more than soap and water. They are likely to become scarce during a pandemic as more people begin using them. Hand washing with soap and water is still very effective when done properly.

The virtue of cleanliness

To help reduce the presence of contagion within the home, keep sick people and their bed and bedclothing clean and dry. The sick rooms and bathrooms need to be maintained in good condition. Ventilation of these areas is important, and if possible, natural light will improve the atmosphere. Soiled garments and bedclothes need to be washed and dried, a task likely to be challenging if there is an interruption of electrical and water service. It will be important to wash these soiled items in hot water using soap and chlorine bleach if possible. Drying these items in the sun takes advantage of the powerful antiseptic effect of ultraviolet light. A good clothesline will be an essential item to have on hand.

Hard surfaces should be wiped clean using soap and water, and then sprayed with 1:10 bleach to water solution and wiped down a second time. Allow the bleach solution to stand on the surface for 30 seconds before removing it to help ensure that all the contagion is eliminated. This technique will effectively remove all trace of infectious viral particles and bacteria from body fluids, vomit, and excrement.

Every caregiver will be exposed repeatedly to the pandemic virus in amounts sufficient to cause infection. Despite this fact, if the bird flu pandemic behaves as expected, only 400 out of 1,000 people exposed will develop symptoms of flu, another 400 will get the flu but have no or only mild symptoms, and

200 won't get it at all. Of the 400 who become ill during a moderate pandemic, one person will die. In the case of severe pandemic I expect as many as 32 out of those 400 may die. Those who do develop infection and recover will be immune from the pandemic strain in the future. All in all, the odds are good that you will survive but not escape the flu. We will all be affected, some more than others, but no one will escape the touch of "the grippe."

Supportive treatment of influenza

It will be useful to keep well-organized notes arranged in chronological order on the patients you are caring for at home. Having a standard approach is a good way to be sure that you have not overlooked anything of importance. Being able to look back at the notes can be a tremendous help when taking care of these patients. Keep an accurate record daily. Each day, start with the patient's vital signs. Include their temperature, pulse rate, breathing rate, blood pressure, and weight if they can stand. Repeat the vital signs three times daily in routine patients and more often in very sick patients. You can get a clear picture of how the patient is doing from these simple measurements.

Home Influenza Treatment

An important part of the daily record is to measure the patient's fluid intake and output. To do this, you will need to record the fluid they are taking in as well as passing out. Intake is easy since you are giving them the fluids, but output can be difficult to accurately record. Have patients save all their urine by urinating in a chamber pot or urinal instead of the toilet. Measure the urine output using a large measuring cup.

The amount of fluid we take in each day is always more than the amount passed out because of *insensible losses*. Insensible losses include fluid lost through the skin as perspiration, water vapor in the breath, and fluid in the stool. If the patient is incontinent of urine, just indicate in the record that the patient was incontinent of a small, medium, or large amount of urine. At least twice each day, add the intake and subtract the output. A rule of thumb for adults is a minimum daily intake of two to three quarts of fluid. Commonly, people drink more than this every day. Fever and diarrhea both increase this basic requirement. If the patient is not getting enough fluid in, their output of urine will fall off, and the urine will become darker and concentrated. If you observe this occurrence, push the patient to drink more fluids.

The SOAP Note method

The **SOAP** medical note format is a useful way to organize medical information on patients.[75] I recommend using this method because it is simple and efficient, yet thorough. "**S**" is for "subjective" and describes what the patient tells you about their illness--how they feel, what hurts and where, what they did for the symptoms, etc. "**O**" stands for "objective" and includes the things you observed or measured. This means vital signs, skin tone, fluid in, and urine out. "**A**" is your "assessment" of the patient's medical condition. "**P**" is the "plan" you make for helping the patient get better. I use this method in my practice and suggest it for your patient notes.

Example Home Care Patient SOAP Note

Patient Name: Mary Smith

Date of Birth: 3-31-1951

Date symptoms first began: January 15, 2007

1-17-07 3:00 PM Initial Note

*Subjective (**S**): Mary became weak and faint today after suffering from muscle aches and pains for the last couple of days. She has trouble standing up without dizziness. She is nauseated and also complains of headache and sore throat. She is urinating but not as much as usual. She has been trying to drink more but has been busy taking care of the sick. She has not been getting much sleep for the last 2 weeks.*

*Objective (**O**): Vital Signs: Temp: 102°F[76], Pulse: 110/min and regular[77], Resp Rate: 22/min[78], BP 100/60[79], Weight: 122lbs*

The skin is pale and mildly moist. Mary looks very tired but is awake and alert. Her mouth is moist. Her urine is dark.

*Assessment (**A**): Flu with mild dehydration and fatigue*

*Plan (**P**): Push fluids (ORS), ibuprofen 800 mg every 4 hours as needed for temp > 101 or pain. Bed rest. Keep track of fluid intake and urine output. Take VS and check hydration, fluid input/output, 4 x daily. Tamiflu 75mg 2 caps once daily with probenecid 500 mg 2 x daily for ten days begun for treatment.*

1-17-07 6:30 PM

***S**) Mary's sleeping on and off. She feels less faint but still dizzy. She is peeing.*

***O**) Temp 100°F, Pulse 90/min, BP 100/60, Weight 123lbs*

Fluid In: 1500 ml[80] ORS, Urine Out: 250 ml

***A**) Flu, improved symptoms, patient still dehydrated but hydration underway*

***P**) Push more fluids. Rest.*

CHAPTER 6

The Signs and Symptoms of Bird Flu

Is it a bad cold or bird flu?

There are several ways to tell the difference between the flu and less severe illnesses. First of all, unless there are other cases of flu around the area, your illness is probably not flu. The chances of your being the first in your neighborhood to contract bird flu are low. When the flu arrives, it will be easily recognizable. The epidemic nature of pandemic influenza will get everyone's attention quickly. The rapidly rising number of new cases will signal the arrival of the strain as clearly as a claxon's wail. Another sign that someone has flu is how sick they get. Flu is much worse than a simple cold or most other infections. The fever and body aches due to flu are often associated with strong shivering. Healthy people sick with pandemic flu will be so ill and weak they will have a hard time getting up out of bed without help.

To sum up, one way to tell the difference between the flu and other infections is that the flu is severe and an order of magnitude worse than what most of us are used to. Colds, bronchitis, sinusitis, ear infections, and sore throat can lay you low but are less severe. Viruses other than flu cause most of these infections with a few due to bacteria.

During seasonal influenza, the most prominent symptoms are fever, cough, sore throat, runny nose, and general aches and pains. These symptoms are common in bird flu as well and are likely to be the most common if this strain completes its human adaptation and becomes pandemic. A hallmark of influenza that separates it from most other regularly encountered human viral infections is severe body aches. Patients feel like they have been run over by a truck or beaten nearly to death. Everything hurts. It even hurts to open your eyes and look around. Flu-related headache also is quite intense. The sore throat from flu is harsh and makes swallowing painful. Coughing can be so severe that patients bruise their breathing tubes, chest wall muscles, and diaphragm. These muscles become very sore making it hurt to take a breath. Heavy coughing can cause headache, sore throat, chest pain, and abdominal pain.

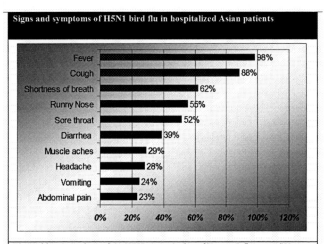

Signs and symptoms of H5N1 bird flu in hospitalized Asian patients

Symptom	Percentage
Fever	98%
Cough	88%
Shortness of breath	62%
Runny Nose	55%
Sore throat	52%
Diarrhea	39%
Muscle aches	29%
Headache	28%
Vomiting	24%
Abdominal pain	23%

The Writing Committee of the WHO Consultation of Human Influenza A/H5., Avian Influenza A (H5N1) Infection in Humans. N Engl J Med 2005;353:1374-85. (Medical References)

The WHO Writing Committee published a 2005 study of bird flu in patients from Southeast Asia in the *New England Journal of Medicine*. [16] Patients who were the subject of this report were so sick they had to be admitted to the hospital. As bird flu evolves to become more infectious for humans, its clinical presentation will also shift, an important consideration when interpreting this information from the early cases in Vietnam. These patients' disease signs and symptoms are presented in the accompanying graph.

The seasonal influenza virus usually enters the body through the respiratory tract, but flu also can gain access through the intestinal tract. Two out of five of the cases presented in the *New England Journal* article had diarrhea, indicating the virus already has the specialized receptors needed to attach and enter the cells lining the human intestine. When the infection begins in the gut, it presents with fever, nausea, vomiting, abdominal pain, and diarrhea. Since so many of the Vietnamese patients reported in the WHO study had gastrointestinal symptoms, ingesting the virus most likely played an important role in their infections.

If H5N1 acquires the genetic sequences necessary to attach to the mucus membranes of the human upper respiratory tree, as seen in seasonal flu, this entry will become the preferred one for the virus. Since the virus already has the ability to efficiently invade and reproduce itself in the human lower respiratory tract (lung), the only thing stopping bird flu from achieving pandemic status now is its lack of receptors for the human nose and back of the throat (pharynx). This hurdle is the last for the virus to cross to cause the next influenza pandemic.

The symptoms people develop with pandemic influenza are more likely to resemble seasonal flu than the presentations seen in these early cases from Vietnam. Most likely, the pandemic virus will infect most people through the upper respiratory tree, where it will cause local symptoms including sneezing and a runny nose. A sore throat, fever, and muscle aches and pains will follow. Over the next day or two, the virus will move into the lower respiratory tract, infecting the bronchial passages and the lung. This will cause cough, more fever, headache, and general weakness. The intestinal presentation will still occur but will be less common.

Several strains of bird flu carry a receptor for the tissues surrounding the brain, allowing the virus to gain access to the central nervous system. This complication is challenging but hopefully rare.

The January 2006 bird flu clusters in Turkey added a clinical feature not previously or since seen: bleeding from the gums and throat. This sign suggests that the virus was able to enter the body though the tissues in the mouth and this may be partially responsible for the large clusters during that outbreak.

Principal symptoms of influenza

Fever

If the patient does not have fever, they probably don't have bird flu. We can expect this symptom to be present in every patient. The virus itself does not cause fever. Rather it is caused by the reaction of our immune system and is one of the ways we fight infections. Virus and bacteria don't grow as well when our body temperatures are higher than normal, and our body's immune system is more active when we have a fever. So, some fever is good for fighting infections. On the other hand, too much can damage and accelerate dehydration. The "best" temperature for balancing the benefits vs. the deficits is between 100.5°F and 101°F taken orally. If taken rectally, increase the range by ½ degree.

Cough

Almost every patient with influenza develops a cough. In fact, if the patient does not have a cough, then there is only a one in eight chance that he or she has bird flu. A wet cough is one that produces phlegm or mucus while a dry one does not. Coughing serves several useful purposes. The most important is to help clear the bronchial passageways of collections of mucus or other debris that accumulate under conditions of health and disease. In this case, cough is helpful. On the other hand, when the cough is not due to the accumulation of mucus or debris but instead caused by irritation on the delicate tissue lining the breathing passageways, then coughing can cause damage. A violent, non-productive coughing spell can bruise the vocal cords and bronchial tubes, causing hoarseness and pain with breathing. The vigorous and intense contraction of the back, abdominal, and rib muscles occurring repeatedly during coughing can bruise or tear them. This leads to pain when taking a breath or when these areas are pressed with the fingers.

Cough was Present in 88% of Asian Bird Flu Patients

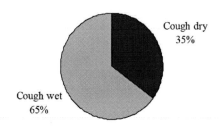

In the Vietnam case studies of bird flu patients, 88% had cough with most being wet rather than a dry one. The dry cough serves no therapeutic purpose and causes considerable damage to the pulmonary structures. In some cases, this damage could contribute to a secondary pneumonia due to the patient with chest and abdominal wall pain suppressing the depth of their breath to prevent intense pain. This leads to accumulation of mucus and bacteria in the lung that would ordinarily be removed if the coughing weren't so painful. The dry cough is the one we want to suppress, and the wet cough is the one we want to encourage.

In patients with infections of the ears, nose, throat, or sinuses, cough can occur when mucus from these irritated tissues finds its way down into the bronchial passageways. Cough from this cause is best treated with an antihistamine and decongestant rather than a cough suppressant.[64,81]

The dry cough is the one we want to suppress, and the wet cough is the one we want to encourage.

Shortness of breath

When a person is *short of breath*, they are having a hard time getting a satisfying breath. They have air hunger. Sometimes this shortness is due an asthma attack or when the air passages go into a spasm of tightening. The patient wheezes when they inhale and exhale breath. The higher the pitch of the wheeze, the more constricted the bronchial tree.

With other causes of shortness of breath, the breathing passages are wide open, and the problem is deep in the lung due to fluid or pus filling up the air exchange area called the *alveoli*. Shortness of breath is one of the hallmarks of severe influenza, and along with dehydration, is one of the common reasons patients with flu are admitted to the hospital for treatment. In the bird flu patients from Vietnam admitted to the hospital, three out of five were short of breath. When a bird flu patient develops shortness of breath during the course of the illness, it suggests they could be developing a complication of influenza. If at all possible, influenza patients having trouble breathing should be evaluated at a hospital.

During the 1918 pandemic a particularly aggressive presentation of influenza pneumonia was seen most commonly in young adults. It was associated with cyanosis, a bluish discoloration of the skin and is described in the following excerpt from a physician's letter to a colleague.

> "After a few hours later you can begin to see the Cyanosis extending from their ears and spreading all over the face, until it is hard to

distinguish the colored men from the white. It is only a matter of a few hours then until death comes." -British Medical Journal, December 22, 1979

Difficulty breathing due to pneumonia and pain when breathing due to a sore chest and abdominal wall are two very different problems that home caregivers need to understand. Both can cause this symptom, but pneumonia is a life-threatening flu complication, while chest wall pain hurts but does not usually affect survival. When a flu patient becomes short of breath, it suggests they may have suffered a dangerous complication of this disease. Whenever this happens, get professional medical help for the patient.

Assessment and remedies for common Bird Flu patient signs and symptoms with a poor prognosis		
Symptom or Sign	Likely Assessment	Remedy
Shortness of breath	Pneumonia, Prognosis Type I or II	Push fluids
Cyanosis (skin turns blue)	Respiratory failure caused by flu pneumonia, ARDS, or secondary bacterial pneumonia. Prognosis poor. Prognosis type 1	Keep as comfortable as possible. Give hydrocodone for comfort & diazepam for anxiety
Bleeding from any orifice and/or severe bruising.	A severe blood clotting disorder due to an overwhelming flu infection (DIC). Rapid death is likely. Prognosis type 1	Keep as comfortable as possible. Give hydrocodone for comfort & diazepam for anxiety

Most people who will die during an influenza pandemic will do so from pneumonia or dehydration. Dehydration can be readily detected and treated at home and explaining how to do that is one of the major focuses of this manual. Pneumonia has such grave implications, it is important that we are able to differentiate pneumonia from simple chest wall pain caused by excessive coughing.

Patients with both causes of chest pain have trouble breathing and pain when they breathe. A wet cough with lots of colored mucus favors pneumonia. Both can have tender chest walls to finger pressure because of their cough. A dry cough favors chest wall pain but does not exclude pneumonia or ARDS. High fever, severe weakness, confusion (*delirium*), and loss of consciousness (*coma*) can be features of pneumonia but not chest wall pain. It is common for bacterial pneumonia (Community Acquired Pneumonia) to develop a few days after the worst of the flu symptoms have passed. If the patient with flu starts getting better but then takes a turn for the worse with a return of their pulmonary symptoms and fever, this presentation favors bacterial pneumonia.

If the patient has symptoms suggestive of pneumonia, a physician should evaluate the patient. The instructions given here are meant for use only as a last resort and in the absence of conventional treatment options. Don't delay having the patient evaluated by a doctor if your hospital or doctor's office is open. Professional evaluation and management is preferable and will give the patient the best chance for survival. However, this option may be unavailable at certain times during the pandemic. If it is unavailable, follow the advice for treatment of pneumonia later in the manual.

Pneumonia usually causes the patient to have a wet cough. The mucus can be thick or thin, and the amount may be moderate to copious. When there is a lot of thick phlegm, the patient may have difficulty coughing and removing the phlegm from the body. The mucus can be white, creamy, tan, yellow, or green in color. It can appear rusty, blood streaked, or bloody. Patients who develop pneumonia during the pandemic are at high risk of dying. Their prognosis can be improved if they have access to treatment in a staffed hospital bed or at the very least begin oral antibiotic therapy at home.

Nausea, vomiting, and diarrhea

Vomiting and diarrhea occur when the virus affects the stomach or small intestine respectively. Vomitus contains water, hydrochloric acid, sodium, potassium, and chloride. In response to infection, the intestines secrete large volumes of water, mucus, sodium, potassium, and bicarbonate that leave the body as diarrhea. Diarrhea is usually a watery brownish fluid with or without the presence of red blood. Both vomiting and diarrhea dramatically accelerate dehydration, especially in the presence of fever. When the intestine is infected and food is eaten, the food cannot be digested well because of how the virus affects absorptive cells that line the gut. This will greatly worsen the diarrhea as undigested food makes its way through the intestine, drawing water from the body.

Water going into the intestine is a normal step in digestion, but since the cells responsible for breaking down the food and absorbing the water are unable to do this, the fluid and food remains in the gut. The mix of fluid and undigested food moves rapidly out of the small intestine into the large bowel where it becomes a banquet for the "good bacteria" that live in our colon. This condition leads to an overproduction of gas and acid by the colonic bacteria. The colon reacts by going into spasm, causing campy pain and worsening diarrhea.

Treatment of influenza

Caring for flu patients is something that almost everyone is capable of doing. The skills needed are the same ones parents use to care for young children or that adult children use to care for elderly parents. Our human bodies are endowed with incredible healing powers. We seek to strengthen and support this power when caring for the ill. For the most part, doctors don't cure illness. The body is the real healer. The physician simply provides support and improves the conditions for the body to do what comes naturally to it. There are really very few modern miracles in medical practice. The human body is the real miracle, and the best treatment in many cases, especially influenza, is to support its inherent healing powers. Most of the advice provided by this book is based upon this simple truth. All you can do is the best you can do. So do that with a satisfied mind. You can't save every patient so don't let a tragic loss prevent you from keeping faith in your ability to help most patients with the techniques found here. You may be their only hope.

The basic goals are to keep the patient clean, dry, warm, and well hydrated. Patients need a soft place to lie down, be comforted, told that they are going to be OK, and reassured that you will be there for them. The most important medical treatment is to make sure they have plenty of fluids. Dehydration must be prevented because it can cause fatality. Keeping the patient hydrated is the best treatment for the flu and the one that is most likely to save lives.

Identification and treatment of dehydration

Preventing dehydration in flu victims will save lives. When patients have a fever, vomiting, and/or diarrhea, they lose much more water from the body than is commonly appreciated. Symptoms of dehydration include weakness, dizziness, headache, confusion, and fainting. Signs of dehydration include dryness of the mouth, decreased saliva, lack of or very small urine volume that is dark and highly concentrated, sunken eyes, loss of skin elasticity, low blood pressure, especially upon sitting up or rising from the sitting to the standing position, and fast pulse rate, especially when moving from the lying to sitting or standing positions.

Preventing or treating dehydration in people with flu will save more lives than any other intervention during an influenza pandemic.

Fever is an especially easy way to rapidly become dehydrated with no one noticing. This happens because of an increase in the normal amount of fluid that leaves the body in the form of water vapor from the skin's surface. The increase is due to the body's need to cool itself by evaporation of water passing through the pores of the skin as perspiration. Since we don't see this loss as it occurs as is the case with diarrhea, it is called an insensible loss. Great quantities of fluid can escape a patient this way. The smaller the body size and the higher the temperature, the faster this can happen. Water in the form of vapor also is lost through the breath. Breathing rapidly is another source of hidden fluid loss.

The ORS formula "A" is excellent for treatment of dehydration from increased insensible losses due to fever, decreased oral intake, and vomiting. If the patient has become dehydrated because of diarrhea, use the alternative ORS "B" formula because with diarrhea, patients lose bicarbonate that is replaced by the baking soda (sodium bicarbonate) in the formula. If they are both vomiting and have diarrhea, alternate ORS "A" with "B" to give a balanced therapy. This adjustment to the ORS will work very well. The ORS formula is slightly different for kids so please refer to the pediatric section for the details.

The Adult ORS formula "A" for dehydration
I-quart clean water
I level tsp table salt
3 tbsp table sugar

The Adult ORS formula "B" for dehydration due to diarrhea
I-quart clean water
½ level tsp table salt
½ level tsp baking soda
3 tbsp table sugar

The quantity of sugar in the ORS can be varied depending on patient preference. It can be increased up to 4 tbsp or reduced to 2 tbsp if desired by the patient. Bear in mind that each table-spoon of sugar has about 60 Kcal of energy. This sugar can be an important source of energy for fasting patients. The sugar provided in the ORS helps spare the breakdown of muscle and organ protein that would occur otherwise, and it is one of the reasons it is included in the formula.

For some people, the ORS will taste too salty. In this case, increase the water content to I.5 or even 2 quarts leaving the remainder of the formula unchanged.

The ORS is really a very sophisticated medical treatment. It is just what the thirsty body needs to restore the lost fluid. It is natural in every respect and the sodium, chloride, and sugar team up to facilitate the passage of water and electrolytes (mineral salts) from the intestine into the blood. You will be amazed at how quickly it revives a dehydrated patient. Plain water is good if that is all you have, but the ORS works faster and better.

If you detect or suspect that dehydration is developing, administer the appropriate ORS fluid by mouth. If the patient is too ill to drink, someone must sit with them and administer the fluids using a teaspoon or the baby bottle to get one spoon full or dribble from the bottle down the patient's throat until she or he is strong enough to drink alone. Don't stop until the patient has been able to keep down at least a quart of fluids, which may take several hours. After the first quart, the patient should become more alert and be able to drink from a glass using a soda straw or a squeeze bottle. They should begin to urinate again. If they are too weak to use a glass and straw or squeeze bottle, try an 8 oz. baby bottle or a plastic squeeze bottle with a squirt nipple, which may be easier to handle than a glass and straw.

You will know you are making headway with the rehydration treatment when the patient becomes more alert and begins urinating, an indication that their fluid deficit is partially restored. While this sign is good, more remains to be done. With sick patients like these, you need to "push the fluids" so don't let your guard down. Your patient will be very tired. Let them sleep for a couple of hours and then get them to drink more fluids. Be insistent; it is really important.

When well hydrated, an adult should pass about two cups of urine with each void. The urine should be light yellow to clear in color. When these signs are present, the patient's fluid deficiency is restored. By keeping good records of your patient's fluid input and output, you can spot dehydration early on by noticing a decrease in the quantity of urine output and the character of the urine that is voided, another reason for keeping good records.

Administering fluids to the sick will be one of the main activities, day in and day out, until the crisis passes. Try to get two to three quarts of ORS in your patient every day at a minimum. Those with high fever or lots of diarrhea may need twice as much. Don't give up or slack off. Make this your most important task.

The ORS will be very refreshing for the patient, and it will quickly revive them. ORS can be served cool or hot depending on the climate, patient symptoms, fever status, and preference. A patient with a high fever should not be given hot fluids because it will raise the temperature further, but if you are not having trouble controlling the fever, then hot fluids can be very comforting. A patient with a sore throat will get relief from a hot beverage. A patient hot with fever might prefer a cool or even cold beverage. If it is cold outside, especially if the patient is cold, use hot fluids.

You can drink the ORS plain or add fruit flavorings or natural herbs like vanilla, cloves, cinnamon, or mint. A number of excellent powdered fruit drink products are available at the grocery store that can be mixed with the ORS. The fruit flavored mixes pre-sweetened with sugar should be considered as pure sugar for the purpose of preparing the ORS. In this case, just reduce the sugar content of the ORS by I tablespoon for I tablespoon of powdered mix used.

Be creative. Jell-O or Popsicles made with ORS, anyone? You can make the ORS substituting fruit juice for water and sugar. Another idea is to use the ORS to make hot beverages for the patient such as tea or hot chocolate.

Once the patient is well hydrated and eating, there is no further need for the ORS. Even if the patient is not eating but can drink and remains well hydrated, you can switch them to one of the other fluids listed for use with the clear liquid diet such as juice, bouillon, or tea.

Assessment and remedies for common Bird Flu patient signs and symptoms with a good prognosis		
Symptom or Sign	Likely Assessment	Remedy
Low urine output	Dehydration	Push fluids
High pulse rate > 90)	Dehydration or fever	Push fluids
Fever	Due to the immune system release of chemicals (interferon, cytokines interleukines,) that fight the infection	Ibuprofen, acetaminophen, push fluids, consider tepid water baths if > 102 F. Treatment goal <101 F.
Shaking chills and shivers	Viremia (virus in the blood) or pneumonia	Keep warm
Sore throat	Direct viral infection of the throat. Pain due to inflammation and damage of tissue in the area.	Gargle with hot salt water; drink hot tea or hot water, use ibuprofen and or acetaminophen.
Cough	Viral infection and irritation of the breathing tubes (bronchial) and/or the lung tissue (alveoli).	Push fluids, drink hot tea DM or hydrocodone cough syrup,
Headache	Due to fever, coughing, or viral infection	Ibuprofen and/or acetaminophen or hydrocodone if very severe
Runny nose	Upper respiratory infection	Use salt & soda nasal wash and diphenhydramine or promethazine antihistamines
Facial pain	Sinusitis complicating flu	Salt & soda nasal wash, antihistamines, azithromycin, pain treatment

Treatment of fever, body aches and pains, and chills

Both ibuprofen and acetaminophen are good ways to lower fever and help the patient feel better. The therapeutic dose of ibuprofen for adults is 2 to 4 tablets (400mg to 800mg) every four to six hours as needed.[82] For acetaminophen, the dose is two 500mg tablets up to four times daily as needed. Try one or the other at the dose recommended. Wait 45 minutes. If the response is insufficient, add a full dose of the other drug. In adults, acetaminophen and ibuprofen can be used in full doses at the same time, because they are in different drug classes and have different drug side effects. Combination treatment with both has an additive effect of benefit without increasing risk. Do not exceed these doses for either drug. This is the maximum for both. Acetaminophen is a very safe drug as long as you do not exceed the daily dose limit for it.

The dose for children and adults is very different. If you are treating a child, refer to the section on using these drugs in children and use the weight or age specific dosing instructions found in the chapter on home compounding of drugs.

Many cold and flu preparations sold in drug stores include acetaminophen or ibuprofen along with antihistamines and or decongestants. These are fine to use for flu. Just remember to include the dose of these drugs in your daily limit calculation to avoid exceeding it for any of the drugs listed.

There is a small risk of causing Reyes Syndrome in children and teens with fever who are given aspirin or aspirin-like drugs including ibuprofen but not acetaminophen. Reyes is a rare occurrence (1:1,000,000 annually) but can be a fatal. Reyes is associated with increased pressure in the brain and liver damage. When confronted with a child or teen with an unremitting high fever (>104°F) who is not responding to acetaminophen, hydration, and tepid water sponge baths, one has to consider the risk of brain damage from fever and seizures versus risk from

Reyes. High fever can literally cook the brain. It is associated with seizures, especially in the very young. The U.S. Government advises against using these ibuprofen-like drugs in children and adolescents.

A high fever (103°F) is hard on the patient, but most folks can tolerate it well. A fever above 104°F is the upper safe limit for most people and anything above 105°F is a temperature emergency. Fevers this high can cause seizures and above this point brain damage can develop if prolonged. This must be avoided. The mainstays of therapy are keeping the patient well-hydrated, tepid water sponge baths, acetaminophen, ibuprofen, and dressing the patient lightly. These treatments used alone or in combination usually work well for a high fever. If the fever resists these techniques and you have access to either ice or snow, you can make a cold pack by placing them in a zip-lock bag and wrapping this up in a kitchen towel. Place a cold pack under each arm, on the right and left sides of the groin, and around the neck. This placement cools the blood as it passes by the icepacks. The head is an excellent place to apply a cold pack too. Another strategy is to sponge bathe the patient and fan them to cool the body by evaporation. Never use alcohol for sponge bathing instead of water. Alcohol can be absorbed through the skin, especially in children, resulting in toxic effects. The goal is to lower the temperature to below 101°F.

Chills cause shivering and lead to contraction of the blood vessels in the arms and legs forcing the blood to the big vessels within the center of the body. The effect is to raise the core temperature to a higher level. When patients have a chill and shiver, they feel cold even if the room is warm and cozy to everyone else. Give them an extra blanket or a hot water bottle to help keep them feeling warm.

Treatment for sore throat, headache, cough, and chest conditions

Gargling with a hot salt and soda water solution is a good treatment for sore throat. To make this treatment, add 1 tsp of salt and ¼ tsp of baking soda to a cup of hot but not scalding water. Ibuprofen and acetaminophen used in full doses either individually or together if needed have good pain relieving effects. If these treatments are inadequate, then add a 2.5 mg of hydrocodone with acetaminophen every four to six hours as needed to the above treatment, remembering to reduce additional acetaminophen each day to stay below the upper limit.

Headache with influenza can come from several sources. Coughing shakes the head back and forth and can strain the neck muscles causing headache. Cytokines released by the viral infected cells and the immune system can trigger headaches. Bacterial sinusitis complicating flu causes facial pain and headache. The treatment of headache begins with treatment of the underlying cause if known. Treatment of the symptom of headache is also appropriate even if the cause is unknown. The use of ibuprofen, with or without acetaminophen, is the first line of therapy. Use 1 or 2 mg of diazepam every four to six hours as needed for relief of neck muscle spasm. An ice pack applied to the neck or head can be a very effective treatment for some patients. The addition of 2.5 mg of hydrocodone with acetaminophen every four to six hours as needed for severe headaches not responding to the prior therapies is the next step.

From the therapeutic standpoint, we want to encourage patients with a wet cough to clear the mucus from their lungs. The health of the patient is unaffected if the phlegm brought up with a wet cough is swallowed or deposited in a handkerchief. Hydrating the patient with the ORS, feeding them a hot or cold caffeine-containing beverage like tea, coffee, or cola, or eating chocolate encourages a wet cough.

The cough reflex is effectively suppressed with dextromethorphan, the drug found in many OTC cough products with the "DM" notation on their label. For a difficult-to-control cough not responding to DM, a 1 to 2 mg dose of the opioid analgesic hydrocodone every four to six hours, is an excellent cough suppressant. If the patient has a wet cough and is coughing a lot, you still should suppress it to prevent the cough from damaging the chest or pulmonary structures. Too much coughing, even when bringing up phlegm, can cause damage and should be lessened.

Chest pain during flu is often due to the effect of coughing on the muscles, ribs, and cartilages that surround and support the lungs. An indication of this cause is when pressing on the chest wall, upper flanks, or upper abdomen brings out the pain. Treatment is to suppress the cough as explained above, allowing these injured tissues to heal. Pain can be controlled using a full dose acetaminophen and/or ibuprofen and 2.5 mg of hydrocodone with acetaminophen every four to six hours. Muscle spasm can play a role in this pain, and when it does, consider adding 1 or 2 mg of diazepam to the mix to lessen this symptom. Chest pain can be excruciatingly painful and require more medication to control. Remember that these medications when used together have greater effects than when used individually. The goal of treatment is not to totally eradicate the symptom. The idea is to reduce it so that the patient is able to rest well and recover.

Inhaling warm humidified air helps patients with infections of the nose, sinus, ears, throat, bronchial pathways, and lungs. During winter, the relative humidity is usually low, a condition that aggravates upper and lower respiratory tract symptoms. Patients will be much more comfortable breathing humidified warm air instead of dry cold air. The warmer the air, the more water it can contain. Warm, moist air sooths the inflamed tissues and assists the body move the mucus through the system and out of the respiratory tree. Drainage is increased, which is beneficial. An electric humidifier is the standard method for adding water to the air, and you should obtain one of these if you don't already have one.

If you are without electric power, add humidity and heat to the air by boiling water on an LP or butane gas camp stove or an LP gas burner. If you are using a woodstove, simply placing a large pan of water on the stovetop will add plenty of humidity to the air. If the air is sufficiently warm, you can use a handheld spray bottle filled with clean water and simply spray a mist into the air of the room. This takes a lot of spraying but works pretty well in a pinch. If you are able to keep the patient's room warm, hanging a wet sheet on a make-shift clothesline located within the room will help increase the relative humidity. You can continue to wet the sheet as needed to keep the humidity high.

Home Humidifiers

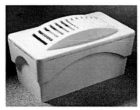
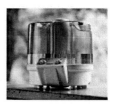

Whole House Humidifier   UV Light Purified Room Humidifier

Food or drink containing xanthenes (tea, coffee, and chocolate) have long been used for treatment of asthma, bronchitis, pneumonia, and chest congestion. They are also very helpful for headache, sore throat, and cough. Xanthenes dilate constricted bronchial tubes, increase the flow of fluid and mucus through the lungs, and stimulate the heart. Blood pressure is raised and more blood is pumped through the body, including the kidneys, promoting urination. The vascular effect of xanthenes relieve headache, and they also have a mildly uplifting effect on brain chemistry that increases energy and alertness. Caffeine is the principal xanthene found in hot or cold coffee and tea. Chocolate products are also loaded with xanthenes. In chocolate, the higher the percentage of real cocoa or cocoa liquor, the higher the content of xanthenes, with dark chocolate having the most. Consuming these foods when ill with flu provides the patient with the pharmacologic effect of their medicinal herbal properties.

Pneumonia following flu that begins at home is called *community-acquired pneumonia* (CAP) to distinguish it from pneumonia that develops in patients while in the hospital. Community-acquired pneumonias have a standard set of bacterial causes, most of which are sensitive to the antibiotic azithromycin, one of the reasons azithromycin was specified in the FTK. There are other choices for treatment of CAP, and I suggest you discuss them with your doctor. All things considered, azithromycin is the drug I recommend first for CAP following flu.

Chest percussion with postural drainage is a technique used to help patients with pneumonia bring up phlegm. Stand by the side of the bed facing the patient. Ask the patient to roll onto their side facing you. Using gentle hand percussion, vibrations are sent through the adjacent lung. Bend over the patient and percuss the patient's back with each cupped hand in an alternating fashion. When correctly performed, there is a musical popping sound produced as air is trapped and slightly compressed between the cupped hand and the patient's back. Repeat this action for three minutes, and then ask the patient to take a deep breath and cough a few times. Administer percussion therapy twice more, then reposition the patient with the other side down and repeat the treatment. The idea is to cause vibrations that travel through the chest wall into the lung and loosen the phlegm, helping move it along the bronchial tree. By laying the patient on their side, you are placing the lung higher than the bronchial tree and using gravity to help move phlegm into the larger bronchial pathways, from where it is more easily coughed up.

Inhaling heated air saturated with water is a time-honored therapy for chest conditions, sinus infection and pressure, ear infections, and sore throat. The easiest way to create steam is by heating water in a teakettle. Once the water is boiling, drape a towel over your head and bend over near but not too close to the jet of steam coming from the spout. Inhale the steamy air through the nose and mouth getting it deep into the lungs.

Steam tents are very effective for children and adults with severe respiratory symptoms from influenza or pneumonia. You can construct a simple steam tent out of inexpensive and commonly available materials using instructions found on the BFM website.

Nasal congestion and sinus pain respond to hot packs placed on the face and by inhaling steamy air. Use of a saline nasal wash to remove mucus and inflammatory chemicals that build up in the nose and sinus also is very useful. Practitioners of Ayurvedic medicine in India first developed this procedure hundreds of years ago. Adding ¼ level teaspoon of table salt plus ¼ level teaspoon of baking soda to I pint of clean water is the formula for the saline nasal wash solution. To use the wash, put about half of a teaspoon of the solution into one nostril and inhale with the other nostril closed. The Ayurvedic tradition uses a device called a neti pot to wash the sinuses, which are handy although difficult to obtain. If unavailable, using a small squeeze bottle or inhaling the solution from a cupped palm or small spoon will serve. An ear-bulb syringe used for infants is another good choice. Inhale and exhale the saline solution though the nostril and then gently blow your nose into a tissue. Repeat the process several times on both sides until air passes smoothly through the nose. Nasal washing can be repeated as often as needed.

If you have access to prescription or over-the-counter anti-histamines and/or decongestants for runny nose or congestion, you can use these products in addition to or instead of nasal washing. Nasal irrigation is the best treatment but the addition of medications can be useful.

Sinus and ear congestion also can be treated with the antihistamines found in the Flu Treatment Kit, diphenhydramine and promethazine. Both products can be given in small oral doses every four to six hours for treatment of nasal and sinus problems.

Treatment of nausea, vomiting, diarrhea, and abdominal pain

The first step in treatment for these four symptoms is to place the patient on type "A" or "B" ORS depending on the presence of diarrhea. The ORS, either administered plain or mixed with a flavoring, is a form of the clear liquid diet. It will not provoke vomiting or diarrhea as easily as other fluids or foods do, but it can still cause these reactions in severely affected people. The drug promethazine works well for control of nausea and/or vomiting. Promethazine can be given orally, by injection, per rectum, and by vagina. In adults, the usual starting dose of promethazine is 12.5 mg every four to six hours by the easiest route tolerated by the patient.

Promethazine commonly causes sedation and a dry mouth. Wait 30 minutes after administration of promethazine for it to begin working. After this period of time has passed, administer a few sips of the ORS to see if the patient can tolerate it. If not, wait another 20 minutes and try again. If the patient still can't take fluids, give her another dose of promethazine and repeat the above steps. The maximum dose of this drug for adults is 50 mg every six hours, but it is very rare to go higher than 25 mg every four hours. The dose of promethazine is the same for all routes of administration.

Assessment and remedies for common Bird Flu patient GI signs and symptoms with a good prognosis		
Symptom or Sign	Likely Assessment	Remedy
Vomiting	Virus affecting GI tract either directly or indirectly	Promethazine for vomiting, push fluids, clear liquid diet
Diarrhea	Virus affecting GI tract either directly of indirectly	Push clear liquid diet, guard against dehydration
Severe stomach cramps	Virus affecting GI tract, probably directly. Expect nausea, vomiting and diarrhea soon.	Hydrocodone and promethazine for comfort, clear liquid diet
Bloody diarrhea without other bleeding.	No other bleeding suggests the patient has the intestinal presentation of Bird Flu.	Hydrocodone and promethazine for comfort, push clear liquid diet

Patients with an intestinal presentation of flu often will experience abdominal cramping, gas, and frequent, loose stools that can irritate the area around the anus. The treatment of irritated skin around the anus begins by *gently cleaning* the area. Use a moistened tissue, soft cloth, or baby wipe. Apply a small amount of petroleum jelly or cocoa butter on and around the anus to protect and heal the tissue. Repeat this process after each loose or normal stool.

Abdominal cramps respond to the anticholenergic effects of diphenhydramine 12.5 to 25 mg every four to six hours and promethazine 12.5 mg every four to six hours. Either of these medications can be tried for this symptom. Using a low dose of the opiate hydrocodone is an effective way to reduce diarrhea and abdominal cramping. Try a dose of 1 to 2 mg of hydrocodone with acetaminophen given every four to six hours as needed for cramps or diarrhea. When an opiate is added to an anticholinergic treatment like promethazine, the effect of both drugs is enhanced on the colon. Therefore, keeping the doses on the small side is best.

Use of opiates for treatment of flu

The synthetic opiate hydrocodone is one of the most effective treatments for a variety of conditions associated with flu. It is approved for treatment of moderate to severe pain and for cough relief in children and adults. In general, the goal with opiates is to use enough to relieve the symptom but not so much that the patient becomes intoxicated or excessively euphoric. It is not necessary to completely eliminate the symptom you are treating with opiates. Rather *control is the goal*. The dose to control a symptom is significantly less than the dose needed to eliminate it altogether. Side effects all increase proportionately with dose, as does the risk of developing tolerance to the beneficial effects of opiates.

Homemade hydrocodone adult dosing guide		
Concentration hydrocodone: 1 mg/tsp		
Symptom	Dose	Frequency
Cough	1 or 2 tsp (1 to 2 mg)	Every 4 to 6 hours as needed
Headache	1 or 2 tsp (1 to 2 mg)	
Muscle aches and pain	1 or 2 tsp (1 to 2 mg)	
Abdominal cramps	1 tsp (1 mg)	
Diarrhea	1 tsp (1 mg)	

Finding the right dose is one of the arts of medicine since people vary in their response to drugs in general and opiates in particular. *Start by giving half the dose recommended in the table and see what the effect is.* The drug takes about 20 minutes to work so give it 30 minutes before giving another ½ dose and see what happens. This treatment should work. If not, give another ½ dose but no more because this much medication is already 50% above the highest dose usually given.

When treating flu-related symptoms such as headache, cough, diarrhea, and abdominal cramps, administer the drug on an as- needed basis instead of a rigid schedule. Flu symptoms vary significantly during the day. By using the opiate only as needed, you may find the patient is comfortable skipping doses or allowing more than the usual amount of time pass between doses. Interestingly, opiates are far more effective if used in low doses infrequently. There is less chance that tolerance to the drug effect of the opiate will develop when used in this way.

Unconscious patients, those with a very sore and swollen throat, or patients with uncontrollable vomiting can still be given medication using the rectal or vaginal route. It is easy to administer medication effectively using one of several simple methods.

The best is to make a simple suppository by mixing the contents of a single capsule or crushed tablet with a small amount of cocoa butter forming it into a small round ball with your fingers. Let this mixture harden at room temperature, place a little cream on the surface of the suppository for lubrication then gently press it into the vagina or rectum of the patient with your finger. The compound will melt rapidly and be easily absorbed, resulting in the desired effect quickly.

Diet and exercise therapy for flu

The flu takes away the appetite, and patients probably won't be hungry. Eating is not as important as drinking fluids because the patient will be breaking down muscle and fat for energy. The *clear liquid diet* is best for patients sick with flu who are not particularly hungry, but it is mandatory for patients with diarrhea due to influenza. If a flu patient wants to eat, feed them as long as they don't have diarrhea. A great deal of water and minerals (sodium, chloride, bicarbonate, and potassium) are lost in the watery portion of the stool with diarrhea, which can lead to dehydration. Patients with diarrhea have to drink considerably more fluids than usual to prevent dehydration. This precaution is especially important if the patient also has a fever, which in itself leads to increased loss of body water through the skin as perspiration. In most cases, patients with diarrhea can tolerate a clear liquid diet without making matters worse. The small intestine can absorb water, minerals, and sugars well even when infected.

If the patient has not been sick long or had a mild non-diarrheal presentation of the flu, you can start with step 2 of the clear liquid diet and quickly move up the steps as tolerated by the patient. At any time during re-feeding, should the patient suffer abdominal problems, especially pain or diarrhea, drop back a step or two on the clear liquid diet. Rest in that step for a while before trying the next step again. This strategy will work well for almost every patient.

The clear liquid diet starts with clear liquids only. As the patient advances through the diet, simple-to-digest, low-residue foods are added one step at a time. Don't advance to the next step until the patient is completely symptom-free in the present step. As the patient progresses through each step, if the cramps and diarrhea return, drop back to the previous step.

The clear liquid diet

- Step 1: Oral Rehydration Solution (ORS), water, fruit juice, Jell-O, Gatorade®, pop cycles, PowerAde®, ginger ale, cola, tea, and bouillon.
- Step 2: To step 1 add white toast (no butter or oils), white rice, and cream of wheat, soda crackers, and potatoes without the skin.
- Step 3: To Step 2 add canned fruit and chicken noodle soup.
- Step 4: To Step 3 add a source of protein like canned meat, fish or egg.
- Step 5: To Step 4 add milk and other dairy products, vegetable oils, butter, raw fruits and vegetables and high-fiber whole grain products.

How to resume feeding patients recovering from flu

If patients have been very sick, especially if the illness has been prolonged, if they have lost weight nor had much to eat recently, you need to be careful when you resume feeding them. Most of these patients will stay in step 1 or 2 of the clear liquid diet during their illness. When you think it is time to resume feeding the patient, move to the next higher step but refrain from rapid advancement through the steps. Give the patient a chance to adjust to each step before moving ahead. Each step may take a day or even two. If you are moving too quickly through the steps, you can rely on the patient's stomach to tell you about it. The signs include abdominal pain, gas, bloating, and diarrhea. Reserve milk and milk products, oils, and high fiber foods until the last step because the digestion of these foods is complex and could overwhelm a flu-weakened small intestine, causing the symptoms above.

Patients whose influenza was characterized by severe diarrhea will have had widespread infection of the cells lining the gut. During the infection, many of these cells were lost as well as the *digestive enzymes* (proteins that break down carbohydrates into simple sugars so they can be absorbed). The body can restore these cells in approximately three days once the infection is cleared, but it can take longer in some patients. When you have a patient recovering from the intestinal presentation of influenza, keep this in mind. Don't try to resume feeding too soon or too aggressively. Any food can cause diarrhea or abdominal cramping.

Once the patient is eating a normal diet without any stomach problems, it is important to increase the intake of high quality protein, especially eggs, meat, fish, or poultry. This nutrition is needed to rebuild the muscle and organ tissue, which were broken down for energy during the illness. Carbohydrates and fats are also important as an energy source for the recovering body and to help replace lost fat stores broken down for energy during the infection.

Exercise during and after recovery

Even moderate influenza causes a breakdown of muscle tissue and physical weakness. If a patient was critically ill with the flu, even more muscle, organ tissue, and fat was broken down by the body for support. While most of us can afford to loose fat permanently, muscle and organ tissue needs to be restored to regain a state of health. Our bodies are designed to accomplish this task with the right diet and graded moderate, regular exercise.

Acute influenza symptoms can be expected to last at least five days but usually seven to 10 days. Most people need another week or two of rest for recovery. A return to limited normal activities is usually possible at this time, but full recovery will not be complete for a month, or even two, after the infection. Of course, no exercise of any type is possible or desirable during the acute phase of the illness. During the recovery period, passive stretching and massage helps a weakened patient recover. These activities help bring the dormant joints, tendons, and muscles back to life and work out the soreness that builds up in these tissues. Gentle passive range of motion (ROM) exercise is accomplished by *slowly and repeatedly* moving all the joints of the limbs, including fingers and toes, through their entire normal range of movement. Each finger and toe, ankles, knees, hips, wrists, elbows, shoulders, and the neck should be bent, rotated, and extended slowly and repeatedly.

The large joints also will benefit from passive stretching after they have been through the ROM exercises. Tendons and ligaments that attach and surround the joints will begin to recover. Perform passive stretching gently using mild hand pressure to extend or flex the joint to the fullest extent tolerated by the patient, holding the stretch for five seconds before releasing it. Repeat three times for each joint in extension and flexion.

After ROM exercise is complete, give the patient a gentle, whole body massage. The idea is to use massage to help remove metabolic byproducts that build up in the muscles and joints when they are sedentary during an acute illness. Begin by gently stroking the major muscle groups of the arms and legs moving from the periphery of the body toward its center. When massaging the torso, move from the waist up to the neck. Massage the head from the crown down to the neck. Stroking the muscles in this manner helps move waste products into the lymphatic channels where they are carried into the blood and broken down by the liver. The patient should be encouraged to drink fluids before and after message to facilitate this cleansing process.

Patients who have been at bed rest for a long time will have trouble with balance and weakness. If they have not been eating, they will not have enough energy to resume normal activity. A prerequisite for getting up is to get the patient past step 3 of the clear liquid diet before even trying to encourage the patient to walk again.

When the time comes to help a patient return to normal, take it easy. Try sitting the patient upright in bed first. If this goes well, the patient can next try sitting on the side of the bed with his feet on the floor. Dizziness and weakness are the two problems that most people have trouble overcoming. Take it slowly. Dizziness usually goes away after a while in the new position, so be patient. The next step is to get the patient up and sitting in a chair. Standing with limited assisted walking comes next. At first, have the patient walk with assistance around the room or in the halls. Then branch out. As strength improves, the patient will get hungrier and stronger. As discussed above, building muscle back requires the consumption of high quality protein. Eggs, dairy, meat, chicken, and fish are the best but not exclusive sources of high-quality protein. You can get complete proteins entirely from vegetarian sources if you know how to mix beans, grains, seeds, and nuts in the correct proportions.

The Zen of being sick

You may become ill yourself. If you have prepared well, then you are not alone and those with you are committed to helping you make it through the illness. Hopefully, you have an adequate supply of medications and materials to assist you and your caregivers during this time. *Remember the most important thing is to drink as much fluid as you can and REST.* You may already be fatigued from preparing for the pandemic. At this point, there is nothing more that you can do, so let it go. Lie down and rest.

Consider being sick as a vacation from the worry, fuss, responsibility, impossible problems, subtle uncertainties, and lack of sleep that sometimes accompany everyday life. Rather than dwell on pain, nausea, and other discomforts, rest assured that you are going to recover. Most people will. Relax. Rest. Let it go. Arrive at the Zen of Being.

When you become ill, withdraw your energies into the quietest place in your being and rest there. The practice is to remain there as an observer or witness. This selfless place is at the heart of each and every one of us--a place of refuge we can access if needed but one most of us seldom visit. Remain there as the observer.

Within this special realm, you are sometimes asleep and sometimes conscious. Your eyes can be open or closed. Time enters a new dimension. Pain and nausea lessen, and you are unafraid. In this place, your mind is free to ride the waves of Being through an inner space.

All our bodies are endowed with the power to heal themselves. Rest is an important requirement for healing to occur. This is the way of life. Your body is able to rest quietly when your mind visits its inner dimension. Abiding within inner space creates the conditions for healing to occur most directly.

Our body's reaction to severe illness or trauma will naturally direct us to this place as long as we don't struggle against it. We have nothing to fear from this old friend. Loosen your grip on reality a little and allow things to slip a little. This letting go can make it easier to move deeper into inner space, an excellent place to ride the dragon. You are not out of touch but rather "not in charge" for the moment. The Zen of Being is a comfortable space where you are not alone and unafraid.

Death and dying

For a small percentage of patients, their health will not improve. When someone dies, a medical professional ideally should confirm the death. If a physician is unavailable, by necessity this task will pass to the next most qualified person. In our contemporary society, it is rare to meet anyone outside the medical profession who has witnessed a death other than that of a family member. Dying and death are entirely natural.

When someone dies from the flu, pneumonia, heart failure, or a massive stroke, the person passes into an unconscious state before death. This *coma* resembles sleep, except the patient is unable to wake from it. The skin of the dying person may feel clammy to the touch. As the dying process unfolds, the body slowly withdraws its life energy from the limbs and concentrates it within the central core. Patients in a pre-terminal coma have withdrawn mentally into a state of deep unconsciousness.

Some patients have abnormal breathing patterns before death, characterized by rapid or deep breathing, followed by a period of no breathing. This process then begins again. This is natural way of the body at the end of life. Some with the "cytokine storm" presentation of bird flu will become rapidly ill and begin to develop a bluish discoloration of the skin that becomes darker and darker over a few hours. Death will follow quickly. We can do nothing for these patients at home and little even in the best ICU. Keep the patients warm and comfortable, assuring them they will not be abandoned and keeping them as comfortable as possible is the only consolation you can give.

When death comes for most people, it will be slow and peaceful. Sometime after the patient enters a coma, breathing becomes progressively shallow and the pulse grows weaker. This pattern can continue for a long time. Close to the end of life, the time between breaths increases considerably. Finally the breathing stops completely. Death has not yet come, but it will inevitably follow in a few minutes.

The person is dead when they have no pulse and no respiration. The dead no longer appear alive. When you see this yourself, you will instinctively know what I mean. If you have a stethoscope, listen for heart sounds in the chest. You should hear no heart or breath sounds. There may be some gurgling from the gut. Listen for a full minute. If after that time you hear nothing, then the person is dead and may be prepared for burial. You also may check for breath by holding a hand mirror near the nose and mouth. When the patient exhales, condensation in the form of vapor can be seen on the mirror. With no exhalation there is no condensation.

CHAPTER 7

Home Care of Children with Flu

Children with flu should not be treated as "little adults". Many differences exist between the way a child and an adult respond to this disease. Many, but not all, of the drugs used for adults are also used for children, but the dose is different. Children have incredible recuperative powers that adult's lack, and a child's immune system is radically different. Despite these differences, some parallels are followed in managing influenza in children and adults. Dehydration and rehydration are critical in both, except that children can become dehydrated much more quickly than adults.

While many of the recommendations and advice for treatment in the other chapters can be applied to kids, some are inappropriate. A wise parent will ask their children's pediatrician for flu management suggestions for use during the pandemic before it begins. You might consider asking the pediatrician to review the suggestions found in this chapter before using them. Your pediatrician knows your child's health better than anyone, and the advice and counsel of your doctor take precedence over any suggestions presented here.

This book is written as a last resort when usual access to medical professionals is unavailable. My recommendations should be considered as general suggestions and guidelines. If you have access to a medical professional and that advice contradicts the recommendations made here, follow your physician's advice. The medical professional on the scene is able to evaluate the child in person and is always best equipped to judge what is wrong and what needs to be done about it.

The solutions suggested in this book for treatment of influenza are designed for use during the extreme conditions expected during the pandemic, not for the ante- or post-pandemic period. So, while many of the suggestions included here may seem impractical compared to the conventional alternatives present during normal times, bear in mind that they are intended for use during emergencies. During the pandemic period, these alternative solutions to common problems will be of greater value.

Signs and symptoms of flu in children

One of the biggest challenges for parents will be trying to tell whether their sick child has a cold or bird flu. If bird flu is not in your community, it is very unlikely that your child will be the first case. One difference is in the speed with which the flu strikes a child compared with a slow-moving cold. All parents know how fast children can go from being completely healthy to very sick. This presentation is common with the flu and less so with a simple cold, which usually develops more slowly over a few days.

Symptoms of influenza in children		
Fever	Fatigue	Loss of appetite
Cough	Headache	Runny nose
Muscle aches	Weakness	Irritability
Sore throat	Nausea	Vomiting
Chills	Ear pain	Crying for no reason
Diarrhea	Dizziness	

Often, the first sign a child is ill will be crankiness or irritability. Usually, this common and non-specific behavior is due to fatigue; so don't jump to any conclusions. Rather, be observant for additional signs. Infants with influenza can suddenly become very sick rapidly or simply "not look right". They may seem unresponsive, dull eyed, and distant. It is not unusual for a runny nose to be followed by a sore throat, and quickly thereafter a fever. Kids with flu will often lose their appetite and have trouble swallowing due to sore throat or swollen tonsils.

How to keep children with flu comfortable[84]

- A child with flu should get lots of rest, which will help her body fight the virus, and keep her more comfortable.
- Use the ORS to provide her with plenty of fluids. Being well hydrated is the easiest way to make nasal mucous thinner, relieve stuffy noses, and soothe sore throats.
- Use a cool mist humidifier in your child's bedroom to reduce coughing, which often gets worse at night.
- Use a nasal aspirator (a syringe that sucks mucus from the nostrils) or ear bulb syringe along with the salt & soda nose spray to relieve stuffy noses in smaller children and infants.

- Older toddlers can be taught to blow their noses.
- For smaller children, raise the head of the crib (with a book or pillow under the mattress) to ease congestion and coughing
- Use acetaminophen for fever, aches, or pains.
- Use a DM (Dextromethorphan) or opioid analgesic (low dose) containing cough syrup to prevent cough[83]

Parents see variations of this scenario repeatedly, especially in the first six years of a child's life. So, when these symptoms develop, keep calm and treat them in the same way you would manage any cold--with fluids, acetaminophen, and rest. Wait to start Tamiflu. Influenza has a special predilection for the respiratory tract, and in most children, it will start in the nose or throat and then spread into the lungs.

If the illness follows this pattern, flu becomes more likely but is still unproven. The feature that makes flu so different from routine childhood infectious diseases is the *severity of the illness.* Kids with bird flu will be very sick very fast. The onset of flu will be easily distinguished from that of a cold. If the child's clinical picture resembles this description, now is the time to start the Tamiflu.

Once the virus moves into their lower respiratory tree, cough develops and the child may become hoarse. Some kids have pain when breathing, which is due to *pleurisy* (inflammation of the covering of the lung). With pleurisy, it hurts to take a deep breath. They also may experience chest wall pain because coughing has bruised the muscles between the ribs and in the abdominal wall.

Dehydration in children

Dehydration presents in children in the same manner as in adults, only more quickly because children do not have as large a fluid reserve. Also, children have a relatively higher skin surface area from which to lose fluids when feverish. The care of children is more challenging because their fluids drop to low levels quickly, especially if diarrhea or vomiting accompanies the fever.

Signs and symptoms of dehydration in children	
Lethargy, reduced movement, fussiness	Decreased urination or dry diapers
Sunken skull "soft spot" fontanel in infants	Tearless crying
Dry mouth or sticky mucus membranes	Sunken eyes
Irritability but may be "too tired to cry"	

Signs and symptoms of dehydration in children

Early in dehydration, a child may be cranky and irritable. Later lethargy or lifelessness may develop. These later symptoms are worrisome signs that indicate the development of dehydration. Begin pushing fluids orally as soon as these symptoms or fever are recognized. The same fluid treatment is indicated for dehydration whether from bird flu or another cause.

If nothing comes of the symptoms, fluid therapy is harmless. Remember to make the administration of fluids as pleasant as possible for the child. If it becomes a punishing or unpleasant experience, the child's cooperation in the future will be compromised, and they may even resist fluids even if their lives depend on it.

When lethargic, children are difficult to arouse. They have very little energy and are "rag doll weak". A child may be flushed or pale with a fever, but if his extremities become cool, severe dehydration has developed and an emergency is at hand. Avoid this situation if at all possible. The heart rate is fast when the child is feverish, but it is also fast when the child is dehydrated. Therefore, heart rate may not help you distinguish the two conditions. A dehydrated child may have a glassy-eyed stare and have difficulty focusing or concentrating. This is never normal and should be considered a sign of the child is very ill and probably needs fluids.

Treatment of nausea, vomiting, and diarrhea in children

The most important treatment for nausea, vomiting, and diarrhea is to stop feeding the child and place them on a clear liquid diet. Use of the appropriate children's ORS is key to preventing and treating dehydration. Nausea and vomiting are treated medically with oral, rectal, or vaginal promethazine in reduced doses as seen in the chapter on Home Drug Compounding. The drug is not approved for use in children under age 2, and in fact serious side effects may occur when used in kids this young. Promethazine will help slow diarrhea and reduce abdominal cramping. It will make the patient sleepy and help lessen a runny nose.

To stop diarrhea, consider using a small dose of the hydrocodone oral suspension. Use a low, age/weight appropriate dose every four to six hours as needed. Recipes for making oral solutions of these drugs are found in the chapter on home compounding along with weight-based dosing guidelines. Nether hydrocodone or promethazine can be used safely in children under age 2. The combination of these two drugs potentates their effects so that 1+1=3. You should begin with smaller than suggested doses of these drugs, especially if you use them in combination.

Another approach for treatment of stomach cramps is the use of a small dose of diphenhydramine oral suspension. The anticholenergic effect of this drug will calm the intestine. Give the child small amounts of the ORS solution in sips from the baby bottle. This will help prevent dehydration and is not likely to make cramping worse.

Treatment of flu in children

Correction of dehydration in children

The principles of rehydration used in adults are the same as for children but the ORS formula is different.

Children's ORS "A" formula for dehydration
1.5-quarts clean water
1 level tsp table salt
4 tbsp table sugar

For kids, use a slightly less concentrated salt solution than with adults. As with adults, the ORS formula for children depends on the source of dehydration. Specifically, if they have dehydration from diarrhea, then use the children's ORS "B". If they are dehydrated due to vomiting or any other cause, then use children's ORS "A".

Children's ORS "B" formula for dehydration due to diarrhea
I.5-quarts clean water
½ level tsp table salt
½ level tsp baking soda
4 tbsp table sugar

If the child is losing fluids from vomiting and diarrhea, alternate ORS formula "A" with "B". As with adults, if the solution tastes too salty for the child, you can dilute it by adding up to two additional cups of water to the formula, and it will still work well.

Treatment of cough

Almost every child with bird flu will cough. As discussed in the adult treatment section, cough has a useful purpose, to help rid the lung of mucus and phlegm. A dry cough is usually due to an irritated bronchial tree, and the more the patient coughs, the more irritated the bronchial tree and larynx becomes. If persistent, the coughing can bruise the lining tissue and vocal cords. These bruises can even ulcerate and become secondarily infected with bacteria.

The trend in pediatrics has been to shy away from use of cough suppressants because of the concern that too much suppression of cough and lung function can be complicated by pneumonia. While a valid concern, a vicious dry cough from bird flu should be tempered to prevent needless damage to the breathing tubes, voice box, and back of the throat as well as the chest, back, and abdominal wall muscles. Caregivers must maintain a fine balance between too much suppression and too little.

Many children will respond well to over-the-counter cough syrups containing dextromethorphan (DM). This drug can cause hallucinations if given for more than several days or in high doses. The opiate hydrocodone is a very effective cough suppressant, but it may cause over-suppression and excessive sedation. One approach is to use DM cough syrup during the day and hydrocodone at night. This way each drug has a chance to clear the system while the other is working. Keeping the child hydrated is very important for treatment of cough.

Another useful technique is humidified air. Using a room humidifier is best but if electrical power is lacking, several alternatives are provided to accomplish this in the section on treatment of adults.

Treatment of runny nose

Rhinorrhea, known more commonly as a runny nose, is a common symptom in children with influenza. The best treatment for runny nose is use of a *salt & soda nose spray* made of ¼ tsp of salt and ¼ tsp of baking soda added to a cup of clean water. It is best to spray the solution into the nose as a mist. One approach is to buy a commercial saline nasal spray at the drug store and use it until it is empty, and then refill it with a homemade salt and soda nasal spray solution. Alternatively, an ear bulb syringe works well for this purpose. The salt & soda nasal stray will help remove mucus and irritants that clog the nasal passage and will help these tissues heal. Use of good nose blowing technique by the child is an important adjunct to successful nasal saline spray use. Using the nasal spray can enhance teaching good nasal hygiene. Again, making it fun and rewarding to use the handkerchief effectively is preferred. Use of positive reinforcement and rewards for a progressive improvement are winning strategies with children. Part of good nasal hygiene is to teach children to wash their hands after they blow their nose or cough into a handkerchief.

Children's salt & soda nasal spray formula
¼ tsp table salt
¼ tsp baking soda
I-cup clean water

Antihistamines are an effective treatment of rhinorrhea in children. Diphenhydramine, the generic name for Benadryl®, is an antihistamine recognized as safe and effective in children. Commercial children's Benadryl is widely available as an oral tablet that melts in the child's mouth. This product is easy to use and a good treatment for runny nose. The Flu Treatment Kit contains diphenhydramine 25 mg capsules. These pills can be formulated into an oral solution for use in children using the recipe and dose table found in the Home Drug Compounding chapter.

Oral diphenhydramine has few side effects other than its tendency to sedate. This side effect actually can be an advantage if the child needs help in sleeping. Sometimes people have an atypical hyperactive response to antihistamines, and if this is the case, they should be avoided, especially in children.

Treatment of fever in children

Children can mount impressive fevers quite suddenly. It is common for fever to go up and down during the day and night. Aches and pains parallel the fever. Fevers can have a daily pattern, and it is common for a child's temperature to reach 104 F during a severe infection. A goal of therapy is to lower the fever to between 100.5°F and 101°F, where the body's immune system is most effective at eliminating invading viruses and bacteria. If the temperature rises above 105°F, seizures or even brain injury is possible. So, it is important to aggressively manage the child's fever before it becomes extreme.

How to take your child's temperature accurately[84]

To measure your child's fever accurately use:
- A rectal or tympanic (ear) thermometer for children less than 3 years old
- A digital (not glass) oral thermometer for children over 3 years old
- Avoid: Using an ear thermometer until your baby is at least 3 months old. It may not be accurate, because young infants have such narrow ear canals.

Temperature readings are different from different parts of the body (rectum, ear, mouth). Your child has a fever if her temperature is above:
- Rectal 100.4°F (38.0° C)
- Oral 99.5° F (37.5° C)
- Axillary (underarm) 98.6° F (37.0° C)
- Tympanic (ear) 100.0° F (37.8° C)

Restoring fluid losses due to fever or other causes is always the first step in treatment of fever. Failure to restore the child's fluid volume will make it nearly impossible to lower the temperature. Acetaminophen reduces temperature and helps with aches and pains. Be sure to use it in full doses rather than partial doses. Use the weight-based guidelines found in the Home Drug Compounding chapter to guide you. A tepid water sponge bath is a useful method in lowering a fever. Never give a child an alcohol sponge bath, which can be toxic. In rare instances, using all the methods above fails to lower the temperature to below 101 F. In this case, lower the temperature of the water you use for the sponge bath or fan the child to speed the evaporation of fluid from the body. An additional measure, if absolutely necessary, is to place ice or snow packs in plastic zip lock-type bags wrapped in kitchen towels under both arms, around the neck, and between the legs on the groin. High volumes of blood are cooled with this technique as it passes by these areas. This method is difficult for the child, but it is a fast way to lower core body temperature in an emergency.

Keeping your child comfortable with a fever[84]

- If the child is shivering, keep her warm until the shivering stops.
- If the child is not shivering, you can remove her warm clothes and encourage her to drink plenty of fluids.
- Keep your child rested, quiet, and comfortable in a cool room.
- Place a cool washcloth on your child's forehead or sponge her with tepid water. Stop if your child starts to shiver.
- Never use rubbing alcohol to cool your child's skin— the vapors are toxic and can be absorbed through the skin.
- Acetaminophen in children's doses is a safe and effective way to lower the fever in kids. It takes from 30 to 60 minutes to begin working.

- Monitor your child's temperature, appearance, and behavior periodically—keep an eye out for signs of a more serious illness—until she seems to be back to normal.

Acetaminophen use in children

Acetaminophen, best known as the brand name product Tylenol®, is an excellent drug for treatment of pain and fever in children from toddlers to teens. It also helps children sleep when given at bedtime. It is very safe with the only issue related to total daily dose, which must not be exceeded to prevent liver injury. In children, the safe dose limit changes with age and weight. The younger a child or the smaller, the lower the safe dose limits. The easiest thing to do is use Johnson and Johnson's brand name Children's Tylenol® or Infant's Concentrated Drops® or the identical generic drugstore brand of these products. If you don't have access to children's acetaminophen, you can make your own using 500mg adult acetaminophen tablets found on the Flu Treatment Kit list. The recipe for compounding this drug is found in Home Drug Compounding chapter, along with dosing guidelines for children. Influenza Drugs

Caution: Opiate use in small children

Hydrocodone, a synthetic opiate, is one of the most effective treatments for a variety of conditions associated with flu. It is approved for treatment of moderate to severe pain and for cough relief in children over 2 years of age only. Children's dosing is lower than adult dosage, and these doses along with guidelines are in the chapter in Home Drug Compounding. The concern with using this drug in children is causing too much suppression of brain and lung function thereby reducing breathing so that secretions might build up and predispose the child to pneumonia. In general, use enough of the medication to relieve but not completely eliminate the symptom. The dose required to relieve the symptom is always considerably less than that required to eliminate it. Side effects increase proportionately with dose. So, use opiates properly and in moderation in every patient, especially in children.

As with adults, start by giving half the dose recommended in the children's dosing table and see what the effect is. The drug takes about 20 minutes to work so give it 30 minutes before giving another ½ dose and see what happens. If the treatment is still unsuccessful, give another ½ dose but no more, because this dosage is already 50% above the highest usually given.

The strategy for treating opiate responsive symptoms during influenza is to use the lowest effective dose as infrequently as possible to control but not eliminate the symptom. When treating the flu-related symptoms such as headache, cough, diarrhea, and abdominal cramps, the doses are given on as-needed basis rather than on a rigid schedule. This flexibility is best because the symptoms in flu can vary significantly. By using the opiate only as needed, patients are comfortable skipping doses or allowing more than the usual amount of time to pass between doses. Opioid analgesics are far more effective if used in low doses infrequently because there is less chance that tolerance to the drug effect of the opioid analgesic will develop. In the Home Drug Compounding chapter, you will find a weight- and age-based dosage guideline for use of this opiate in children as well as a recipe for a homemade oral suspension.

Tamiflu for children with bird flu

Don't begin Tamiflu treatment in anyone until you are sure they have the flu. The reason for holding back is to protect short supplies of the drug and avoid wasting valuable doses when unnecessary. Additionally, research studies on Tamiflu for seasonal flu found that it was ineffective if given more than 48 hours after the onset of flu symptoms. Therefore, you have a treatment window within which you have to decide if the child has influenza or not.

In kids, Tamiflu is dosed on the basis of weight.[54] Roche makes a powder form of the drug that requires the addition of clean water to make a suspension for use in children. If you purchase Tamiflu for children and you plan to buy it in the suspension form designed for kids, please remember to tell the pharmacist not to mix the powder in the bottle with water. Once mixed, the drug will quickly deteriorate. The pharmacist will give you the powdered drug in a single dose bottle for you choose to mix it with water yourself along with instructions for mixing it.

Probenecid, included in the Flu Treatment Kit, is a Tamiflu dose multiplier. When you take it two times a day at the same time you are taking Tamiflu, the blood level of Tamiflu is doubled, and the time it stays in the body is increased 2.5 times from eight hours to 20 hours on average. Probenecid is commonly used in children and even infants to increase levels of antibiotics for treatment of infectious diseases like malaria and bacterial meningitis. [60,61] The doses of probenecid used in children for this purpose range from 25 mg to 40 mg per kg per day given in a twice-daily dose. In the chapter on Home Drug Compounding, you will find a dose guide for use of probenecid in children based upon body weight.

Although Tamiflu-resistant influenza is a possibility, the drug should still be used for treatment of bird flu in children.

Tamiflu resistance is common especially in children who have seasonal flu. The flu has to partially cripple itself to become resistant, and the crippled virus is less likely to cause serious illness than unaltered virus. In my opinion, this development may actually turn out to be a positive.

CHAPTER 8

Home Treatment Guide for Medical Professionals

This section of the book guides health professionals who will be training lay caregivers, supervising their work, and providing routine and advanced direct patient care in the home setting. Some of the procedures in this chapter could harm patients if used improperly. Therefore, the suggestions in this chapter should be reserved only for trained health professionals. In the Advanced Home Treatment section of the website Resources, I have placed several additional articles about treatment of flu. Unfortunately, most of the published information is written for use in the hospital or clinic environment using techniques and methods exclusive to those treatment settings. There are some materials written for use under austere or wilderness conditions that have application to a pandemic scenario and I have placed them on the website for the use of healthcare professionals.

Leading the home care effort

A severe pandemic could cause a temporary disruption of the traditional delivery of healthcare services. In this case, medical personal employed in health care facilities most likely will be at home with their families. Many people ill with flu will have to cope with this illness at home. Some may be alone, and more than a few could be desperate for help. Health professionals will have a unique opportunity to work together in ad hoc neighborhood health networks formed to serve families, friends, and neighbors during the pandemic.

A reasonable first step in addressing the medical needs of your neighbors is to identify how many health professionals live nearby and what medical skills they possess. By pooling the talents of the available health professionals and working as a team, you will be able to accomplish much more than if working individually. While the medical team will be unable to assume direct patient care of everyone that needs it, it can assist family members, friends, or neighbors to provide the bulk of patients' care. For the most part, this activity means supervision as well as providing advanced techniques and methods when needed.

Once the medical team is assembled, it is necessary to take an inventory of the medical resources in the neighborhood. If you have the foresight to form your team before the pandemic begins, consider establishing an essential medical supplies stockpile that includes key pharmaceuticals. If your network forms after the pandemic has begun, there may still be time to obtain the needed supplies in the conventional manner. If not, it's time to scrounge. Methods of adapting many commonly available items found in drug, hardware, and auto parts stores for medical purposes are provided here and on the BFM.com website. By being imaginative and resourceful, you will be able to adapt common everyday items for medical purposes. So, keep your eyes open.

While this manual focuses exclusively upon influenza and its management during pandemic conditions, health care providers also will confront the medical needs of patients with other minor and serious conditions during the course of a pandemic. These needs will range from poison ivy to myocardial infarction. For instance, psychiatrists may be called on to deliver a baby or the internist to remove an appendix. In the event of a collapse of the conventional delivery system, the diagnosis and treatment of these conditions will fall upon your shoulders, irrespective of your ability to manage the situation. I have located some written resources that will be invaluable should your team be confronted with issues that lie outside your skills but for which you remain the best-qualified person to deal with them. A selection of these resources and texts are on the BFM website. Some of the materials are PDFs that can be downloaded for free. Reference books and textbooks as well as additional background material may be well worth purchase.

An aid station within the neighborhood where select patients requiring advanced care can be treated is a good idea. However, no one should think of the aid station as a hospital. Consider having the patient's family or friends bathe, feed, dress, get water for, and clean up after the one being treated in the aid station just as they would in their own home. The purpose of the patient staying in the aid station is to make it easier for you or other members of your team to be able to keep a close eye on the person during the critical phase of his illness and to facilitate administration of advanced treatment options including those listed here as well as your own strategies.

Establish clear guidelines for your neighbors on what they can and cannot expect from your medical team. Draw firm boundaries and stick to them. If you fail to do so, your aid station could become overwhelmed. Also, remember that the head of your team decides who to admit to the aid station, not the patient or the patient's family.

Plan to treat every patient with the same basic level of care, defined here as "good home care". This care is characterized by keeping the patient well hydrated, clean, warm, dry, out of pain, and emotionally comforted. Basic care as outlined here serves the same purpose as hospice care.

Administering fluids to unconscious patients

Nasogastric tube

A low tech and satisfactory way to provide oral hydration to an unconscious patient is via a nasogastric tube. If you are unable to obtain one of these medical devices, consider crafting one by adapting a ¼" outer diameter small polyethylene plastic tubing (available at hardware stores and sold to supply water to a refrigerator icemaker). Administering fluids by NG tube requires some skill and equipment. This equipment, other than the small tube, can be obtained from most major drug chain stores. For instance, a combination douche/enema kit when combined with the small polyethylene tube and duct tape provides all the parts necessary to make a functional NG administration set.

Colonic rehydration

Another way to rehydrate unconscious patients is through the colon.[85] While this technique is not used commonly in the West, many third world countries frequently rely on it. The WHO recommends colonic rehydration as an alternative to oral or IV rehydration when the later options are not available or inadvisable. The colon routinely absorbs fluids and electrolytes from the fecal matter that traverses it.[86] On average, the colon removes 1.5 quarts from the stool each day. While the right colon is better at fluid absorption than is the left, both sides are quite capable at carrying out this function. The WHO suggests using a mildly hypotonic solution compared with standard ORS to enhance fluid and electrolyte absorption from the colon. Since glucose is not normally presented to the colon, and its presence there would cause gas and acid production by the normal bacterial inhabitants of this organ, sugar also has been deleted from the colonic rehydration solution (CRS) formula.

In dehydrated patients, the colon can absorb considerably more volume than 1.5 quarts, but those who have used this technique for rehydration suggest that it is best not to exceed 1.5 quarts of fluid per day.[87] One interesting feature of using this route of fluid replacement is that once the patient's intravascular volume has been replaced, the colon will not absorb additional excess water. This fact could be useful when administering fluids to a patient with congestive heart failure. Obviously if the patient is having diarrhea, rehydration by this route would be inadvisable.

Colonic rehydration solution (CRS) formula
1.5 quarts clean water
1 level tsp table salt

The same administration sets specified for NG tubes will work well for colonic rehydration. Using a permanent black maker pen, mark the end of the tube you plan to place in the rectum every inch up to 12 inches. Place the patient on her left side with her left leg outstretched and the right knee bent. The anatomy of the rectum and sigmoid colon requires that the patient be placed in this position when you are administering fluids rectally. Slowly administer the CRS fluid at a rate of about 250 cc (1 cup) over 1 hour. Faster administration that distends the colon will cause the patient to feel uncomfortable. Then unplug the tube from the bag and clamp the end. Tape this to the patient's leg. Wait 4 hours and then repeat. The adult colon can easily absorb about 1.5 quarts of CRS every 24 hours. For children, the amount of fluid to instill should range from 2 oz (60cc) for infants every 4 hours to the full 250cc for teens weighing 145 lbs or more.

Maintain the left lateral Sims position for an hour, or at most two, after administration of the CRS to provide plenty of time for the fluid to be absorbed. All fluid absorption takes place in the colon with none occurring in the rectum.

Restraining patients

Three-point restraints using cotton sheets cut in lengths is the most humane way to keep a delirious patient in bed and to prevent them from pulling out their NG tube. Consider placing the patient requiring restraint on a twin-sized bed, which is more suited to restraints than a larger bed. To make restraints, cut a cotton sheet into 4'-long 4"- wide strips. Fold the strips over to make 4' x 2" strips. Both wrists and one ankle are restrained using the three-point method. Make sure that the patient is able to move around as much and as easily as possible consistent with your need to restrain them. Tight restraints should be avoided.

A waist restraint is an effective way to keep a delirious patient in bed when you are unconcerned with the patient pulling out an NG tube. This restraint also can be fashioned from a bed sheet. Cut the sheet along its long axis into a 48"-wide strip.

Fold the strip to obtain a 12" width. You may wish to sew the strip together at this width to keep it from coming undone. You also may need to sew two strips together along the long axis to obtain a sufficient length to properly secure the restraint to the bed. Loosely wrap the folded sheet once around the patient's waist and secure both loose ends to the sides of the bed frame. This method will keep most folks in place--except the wigglers who somehow manage to do the limbo right onto the floor. They may require three-point restraints.

The waist restraint also is effective for assisting a confused elderly person in sitting upright in a comfortable chair.

Tamiflu treatment and resistance

The effective use of Tamiflu may be different during pandemic conditions compared with seasonal flu. Until more is known, consider starting Tamiflu in every patient in whom it might help, no matter how long they have been sick. Active viral reproduction is occurring in these patients, and Tamiflu may be of help in speeding their recovery. If you have access to Tamiflu, the dose for seasonal flu is one tablet twice daily for 5 days. Studies have found that in seasonal flu Tamiflu works best when started within two days of the beginning of symptoms. Almost no information on how to use Tamiflu for treatment of bird flu exists although we have hopes that the Chinese, Indonesians, and Vietnamese will soon be publishing their experience with the drug. This research will provide important guidance on the optimal dose and length of treatment needed to obtain the best patient outcome. I will be providing updates on the BFM.com website as they become available. <u>Medical References</u>

Since the Tamiflu-resistant strains are less lethal than the Tamiflu-sensitive ones, use this drug even when Tamiflu-resistant strains are circulating makes sense. The strains which are sensitive to it, and which the drug eliminates, are much more lethal than the resistant ones. If the strain you are treating is Tamiflu-sensitive, great. The Tamiflu will help. If not, the outcome is still be better than without Tamiflu. The patient is infected with a lower risk strain of bird flu and employing the Tamiflu in him prevents the emergence of the more lethal coexisting Tamiflu-sensitive strains.

Are higher Tamiflu doses and longer treatment courses needed?

At the present time, public health and infectious disease professionals are debating whether to raise the dose and length of treatment. One regimen under consideration for treatment of pandemic influenza in adults is two 75 mg Tamiflu capsules twice daily for 10 days. By doubling the dose and time of treatment, the quantity of drug required increases by a factor of 4. A severe shortage of Tamiflu may make it politically impractical for any official body to recommend higher doses of the drug to be used for treatment. As the pandemic approaches, this controversial issue will surely become even hotter.

Co-administration of Tamiflu with Probenecid

One possible solution to the Tamiflu shortage first suggested by Joe Howton, MD, Medical Director of the Emergency Department at Adventist Medical Center in Portland, Oregon, is combining Tamiflu with probenecid.[88] The plasma level of Tamiflu is doubled and the half-life increased to 20 hours from

8 hours by the co-administration of probenecid.[59,62] Using this combination boosts the effective stockpile of Tamiflu by a factor of at least 2.5. To obtain the benefits of this combination, probenecid should be given in a dose of 500 mg by mouth 2 times daily in adults with a lower dose for children. Doing so safely reduces renal excretion of oseltamivir carboxylate, the active metabolite of Tamiflu by 60%, doubles the plasma concentration, and increases the half-life by 2.5 times. Overall, the area under the receiver operator curve is increased by 2.5 times that of the same dose without probenecid. In clinical trials of Tamiflu given at higher doses, no significant increases in side effects or any new or dangerous side effects occurred.

One of the most important benefits children and adults have from the use of Tamiflu for treatment of the flu is reduction of the chance of suffering a complicating secondary bacterial pneumonia, bronchitis, ear infection, or sinusitis. This feature is associated with a reduced need for both use of antibiotics and hospitalization after influenza. Tamiflu does not appear to prevent the development of cytokine storm in adolescents or young adults.

Urine and the management of dehydration

Diagnosis of dehydration objectively with urine specific gravity (SG)

Urine specific gravity is best measured using a *hand-held refractometer*. You also can use a urine dipstick to estimate SG. Urine SG is an excellent objective measure of the state of a patient's hydration given normal renal function. Urine SG ranges from 1.000 (distilled water) to 1.035 (really concentrated). Normal kidneys can easily concentrate urine to 1.020 or above without difficulty after a typical overnight fast. Patients with chronic renal insufficiency are unable to concentrate urine much above 1.010. A clinically dehydrated patient with a urine SG of 1.010 is diagnostic of renal failure. To use SG to manage the patient's fluid intake is simple. Assuming that the patient has normal renal function, all you need to do is adjust the rate of oral fluid administration to maintain the urine SG between 1.010 and 1.020. A refractometer can be costly. However, devices manufactured for veterinary use have the same technology as those designed for humans and cost considerably less.

Estimating the state of hydration based upon urine characteristics

In patients with fever, urine is usually concentrated, reflecting the patient's dehydrated state. You can accurately measure urine concentration directly with a urine refractometer or a dipstick that includes a measure of specific gravity. Since these tools may not be at your disposal, the next best methods are those employed by practitioners of the forgotten medical art of uroscopy.[89] The concentration of urine is estimated based upon its color, appearance, and feel. In the absence of liver failure, hemolysis, hematuria and myoglobinuria, the color of urine is an excellent guide to its concentration: the darker the urine, the more highly concentrated. As for solute content, urine with a high content of visible solute is more concentrated than urine without. The uroscopist holds a clean glass vial of freshly voided urine in a beam of sunlight to determine its concentration. The uroscopist also considers the feel of freshly voided urine. Dilute urine feels like water whereas concentrated urine has more substance, or weight.

In general, the rule is to increase ORS fluids to patients until they begin passing dilute urine. At this point, the patient is rehydrated. You may now continue fluid administration at a maintenance level, paying careful attention to the urine for any signs of recurring dehydration. Since some guesswork is involved, using the uroscopist's method will help you. Obviously, you will need to increase ORS administration when the urine is concentrated. If thirsty, the patient should be encouraged to drink fluids in addition to the ORS. As the patient improves and begins drinking freely, then the need for monitoring the urine character will become unnecessary.

Good medical records

Encouraging the use of simple, but good, medical records will be of great benefit to the patient and the medical professional trying to figure out what is going on with a patient that has taken a turn for the worst. Having this information recorded in a logical fashion, like the SAOP Note, is my recommendation as it is easy to teach to laypersons and sufficiently comprehensive.

CHAPTER 9

Home Drug Compounding

Notes on compounding drugs into suspensions

It is simple to turn drug tablets or capsules into oral suspensions. The skills are the same as those needed to make good biscuits. In fact, baking is more difficult than compounding. To successfully compound tablets or capsules into suspensions, you need to follow a recipe and use measuring spoons and a measuring cup.

Forget compounding, use a pill cutter instead

Physicians can prescribe the drugs for flu as tablets for adults and most adolescents. However, in some cases, a full dose of medication may be too much, even for an adult. To help you divide tablets, purchase a pill cutter from the drug store. They cost approximately $5.00 and will make the task of accurately dividing tablets much easier. For infants and children, the doses recommended are always smaller, and while it is possible to cut or divide tablets or capsules in halves and quarters for kids, this division is difficult to do properly. Additionally, this method is somewhat unappealing for the child. Certainly for children and possibly for use in adults, I suggest you consider compounding your own drug suspensions for treatment of bird flu.

U.S. FDA "approved" vs. "unapproved" or "off label" drugs

While most of the uses that I recommend for the drugs listed in the Flu Treatment Kit are consistent with the U.S. FDA-approved indications, there are exceptions. In prescribing rules and regulations, the FDA gives physicians great latitude to write prescriptions for "off label" indications as long as the physician determines such use is safe and the patient is likely to benefit as a result.

You will need to obtain prescription drugs from your doctor. I suggest that you show your doctor the list and quantities of drugs from the FTK and seek his or her opinion about their use for the treatment of influenza and its complications. Your doctor, who knows your medical history and the other medications you take, may recommend that you avoid one or more of the medications on the FTK list and use a substitute. As previously stated, your doctor's advice trumps that provided here.

Drug expiration dates and compounding

Drug manufacturers are required to place an expiration date on the drug container. The expiration date is usually *always conservative;* meaning that many drugs are good for some time after the printed date expires. The life of a pharmaceutical remains viable particularly when the medicine is stored in the original packing away from sunlight, within the proper temperature range, and at low humidly. If maintained in this way, the drugs in the FTK will last for years after their expiration date and be safe to use and effective. For instance, Tamiflu is stable for 5 years after manufacture when stored properly. Once the container is opened and the product is exposed to air, sunlight, and humidity, then deterioration slowly begins. Compounded drugs, by contrast, spoil quickly. Therefore, if you decide to compound your own drugs into suspensions, don't mix up more than you can use over a month at a time. The quantities that I have recommended are generally those that will be adequate for this purpose.

Preservation of compounded suspensions

Spoilage is due to the contamination of compounded suspensions with bacteria, fungi, and mold. The alcohol ethanol and common table sugar are two natural preservatives with several favorable attributes. This natural preservative is widely available and inexpensive. Ethanol is found in alcoholic spirits as well as made normally in the body during metabolism. The body is designed to handle it easily in small quantities. The formulas provided here use common 190-proof grain alcohol sold in the liquor stores. These formulas assume this ethanol source as the one most easily available during a pandemic. Please note that common rubbing alcohol (isopropyl alcohol) is poisonous and must never be taken orally under any circumstances.

Table sugar also has antimicrobial properties when dissolved in solution at high concentrations. The concentration is the key. When you add the quantity of sugar to the amount of water found in each of the suspension recipes, the concentration of individual sugar molecules is so high that microorganisms can't grow easily in it.

Taste, flavor, and palatability

When compounding a homemade suspension, consider flavoring it with a powdered fruit drink product. Some examples from the Kool-Aid® line of unsweetened soft drink mix include Tropical Punch, Strawberry, Lemon-Lime, Lemonade, Grape, Berry Blue, and Black Cherry. These mixes are free of sugar and artificial sweeteners and sold in individual packs with enough to make two quarts . Alternatives to using the powdered flavorings are herbs like mint or other natural flavors such as lemon or lime juices. Ethanol also affects taste so that when it is added to a drug suspension, it disguises the drug dissolved in it.

Keep out of reach of children

Because these recipes are tasty, some children might drink too much if they are unsupervised. Overdose with either the acetaminophen suspension or the hydrocodone with acetaminophen suspensions are two solutions that are particularly dangerous. Please don't leave any drugs where children or animals can reach them.

Additional information about these drugs

On the Resource Section of the BFM website I have placed the Physician Desk Reference write-up on each of the prescription drugs listed in the Flu Treatment Kit and this chapter on home compounding. The pharmaceutical companies call this document the drug's "product circular" (PC). A good bit of research information is published in the PC along with potential and actual side effects of each drug and safety warnings. I have also placed articles from medical journals that discuss the use of these drugs. Influenza Drugs, Medical References

Tamiflu®

Indications and usage

TAMIFLU is indicated for the treatment of uncomplicated acute illness due to influenza infection in patients one year and older who have been symptomatic for no more than two days.

Children's Tamiflu dosing

TAMIFLU is not indicated for treatment of influenza in pediatric patients younger than one year. In kids, we base the dose for Tamiflu on weight. Roche makes a powder form of the drug that requires the addition of clean water to make a suspension for children. The pharmacist will give you the powdered drug in a bottle, and you will need to mix it with water yourself. A more cost effective alternative is to buy the adult dose of Tamiflu, 75 mg, and use it to make your own children's suspension.

Homemade Tamiflu Oral Suspension for Children

Formula

- 1/2 cup of clean water (125 cc of clean water)
- Tamiflu 75 mg capsules # 5 (five capsules of Tamiflu = 375 mg)
- 1 tbsp sugar
- 1 tbsp grain alcohol (15 cc of 95% ethanol)
- 1/4 tsp flavoring

Recipe

Mix the water, sugar, ethanol, and flavoring in a lightproof container with a good lid. Pour the contents of the capsules into the container, replace the lid, and shake vigorously. Label the container. Store in a cool, dry, and dark place.

Suggested label

- Homemade Tamiflu Children's Suspension
- KEEP OUT OF REACH OF CHILDREN

- Concentration: Tamiflu 15 mg per tsp
- Date formulated: _____
- Compounded by: _____

Children's Dose

See chart: *Guidelines for use of homemade Tamiflu oral suspension in children*

Guidelines for use of homemade Tamiflu oral suspension in children				
Concentration: Tamiflu 15 mg/tsp				
Lbs	Kg	Tamiflu dose in mg given twice daily	Dose	Frequency of dose
15	7	30	2 tsp	Twice daily
21	10	30	2 tsp	Twice daily
27	12	30	2 tsp	Twice daily
33	15	38	2 ½ tsp	Twice daily
39	18	38	2 ½ tsp	Twice daily
45	20	45	3 tsp	Twice daily
51	23	45	3 tsp	Twice daily
57	26	45	3 tsp	Twice daily
63	29	45	3 tsp	Twice daily
69	31	75	5 tsp	Twice daily
75	34	75	5 tsp	Twice daily
81	37	75	5 tsp	Twice daily
TAMIFLU is not indicated for treatment of influenza in pediatric patients younger than 1 year. Source: Adapted by Dr. Woodson from Roche product circular				

Acetaminophen

Indications and usage

Acetaminophen is used to lower temperature and treat pain from any cause. When used according to these guidelines, the drug is safe and effective for these indications and has a low side effect potential.

Safe acetaminophen dosing in children			
Age (Yrs)	Wt (lbs)	Dose (mg)	Daily Limit (mg)
0.1	5	25	100
0.3	10	50	200
0.6	15	75	300
1	20	100	400
2	30	180	720
3	35	180	720
4	40	240	960
5	45	240	960
6	50	320	1280
7	55	320	1280
8	60	320	1280
9	65	400	1600
10	70	400	1600
11	75	480	1920

Homemade Small (< 40 lbs) Children's Oral Acetaminophen Suspension

Formula

- 1 cup of clean water (250 cc of clean water)
- Acetaminophen 500 mg # 5 (five acetaminophen tablets = 2500 mg)
- 2 tbsp sugar
- 2 tbsp grain alcohol (30 cc of 95% ethanol)
- ½ tsp of flavor

Recipe

Mix the water, sugar, ethanol, and flavoring in a lightproof container with a good lid. Add the acetaminophen tablets and give them time to dissolve. Use a blunt end of an unsharpened pencil to crush any remaining fragments. Tighten the lid and shake well. Label the container and store in a cool, dry, and dark place.

Suggested label

- Homemade Children's Oral Acetaminophen Suspension
- DANGER: KEEP OUT OF REACH OF CHILDREN
- Concentration: acetaminophen 50 mg per tsp
- Date formulated: _____
- Compounded by: _____

Children's Dose

See charts: *Small (< 40 lbs) Children's Oral Acetaminophen Suspension* and *Safe acetaminophen dosing in children*

Homemade Oral Acetaminophen Suspension Small Children under 40 lbs					
Concentration acetaminophen 50 mg/tsp					
Age (Yrs)	Wt (lbs)	Dose (mg)	Daily Limit (mg)	Dose	Frequency of dosing
0.1-0.2	5-9	25	100	½ tsp	4 times daily
0.3-0.5	10-14	50	200	1 tsp	4 times daily
0.6-0.9	15-19	75	300	1 ½ tsp	4 times daily
1-1.9	20-29	100	400	2 tsp	4 times daily
2-2.9	30-34	180	720	2 ½ tsp	4 times daily
3-3.9	35-40	180	720	2 ½ tsp	4 times daily
Source: Dr. Woodson, adapted from the Tylenol product circular					

Homemade Children's (> 40 lbs) Oral Acetaminophen Suspension

Formula

- 1 cup of clean water (250 cc of clean water)
- Acetaminophen 500 mg # 20 (20 acetaminophen tablets = 10,000 mg)
- 2 tbsp sugar
- 2 tbsp grain alcohol (30 cc of 95% ethanol)
- ½ tsp of flavor

Recipe

Mix the water, sugar, ethanol, and flavoring in a lightproof container with a good lid. Add the acetaminophen tablets and give them time to dissolve. Use a blunt end of an unsharpened pencil to crush any remaining fragments. Tighten the lid and shake well. Label the container and store in a cool, dry, and dark place.

Suggested label

- Homemade Children's Oral Acetaminophen Suspension
- DANGER: KEEP OUT OF REACH OF CHILDREN
- Concentration: acetaminophen 200 mg per tsp
- Date formulated: _____
  Compounded by: _____

Children's Dose

See chart: *Homemade Children's (> 40 lbs) Oral Acetaminophen Suspension* and *Safe acetaminophen dosing in children*

Homemade Oral Acetaminophen Suspension for Children Over 40 lbs					
Concentration acetaminophen: 200 mg/tsp					
Age (Yrs)	Wt (lbs)	Dose (mg)	Daily Limit (mg)	Dose	Frequency of dosing
4	40	240	960	1 tsp	4 times daily
5	45	240	960	1 tsp	4 times daily
6	50	320	1280	1 ½ tsp	4 times daily
7	55	320	1280	1 ½ tsp	4 times daily
8	60	320	1280	1 ½ tsp	4 times daily
9	65	400	1600	2 tsp	4 times daily
10	70	400	1600	2 tsp	4 times daily
11	75	480	1920	2 ½ tsp	4 times daily
12	90	480	1920	2 ½ tsp	4 times daily
13	95	640	2560	1 tbsp	4 times daily
Source: Dr. Woodson adapted for the Tylenol product circular					

Hydrocodone

Indications and usage

Pain and cough suppression

Off-label uses

Bowel anti-spasmodic, Anti-diarrheal, and sedative

Homemade Children's (>40lbs) Oral Opiate Suspension

Formula

- 1 cup of clean water (250 cc of clean water)
- Hydrocodone 5 mg with acetaminophen 325 mg # 10 tablets (Ten Hydrocodone 5 mg with acetaminophen 325mg tablets = 50 mg hydrocodone and 3250 mg acetaminophen)
- 2 tbsp sugar
- 2 tbsp grain alcohol (30 cc of 95% ethanol)
- ½ tsp of flavor

Recipe

Mix the water, sugar, ethanol, and flavoring in a lightproof container with a good lid. Add the hydrocodone tablets and give them time to dissolve. Use a blunt end of an unsharpened pencil to crush any remaining fragments. Tighten the lid and shake well. Label the container and store in a cool, dry, and dark place.

Suggested label

- Homemade Children's Oral Opiate Suspension
- DANGER: KEEP OUT OF REACH OF CHILDREN
- Concentration: hydrocodone 1 mg and acetaminophen 65 mg per tsp
- Date formulated: _____
- Compounded by: _____

Children's Dose

See chart: *Homemade Children's Oral Opiate Suspension*

Homemade Children's Oral Opiate Suspension				
Concentrations: hydrocodone 1 mg/tsp and acetaminophen 65 mg/ tsp				
Age (Yrs)	Wt (lbs)	Hydrocodone dose in mg	Acetaminophen dose in mg	Maximum Dose
2-2.9	30	0.5	33	½ tsp every 4 hours
3-3.9	35	1	65	1 tsp every 6 hours
4-4.9	40	1	65	1 tsp every 6 hours
5-5.9	45	1	65	1 tsp every 4 hours
6-6.9	50	1	65	1 tsp every 4 hours
7-7.9	55	1.5	100	1 ½ tsp every 6 hours
8-8.9	60	1.5	100	1 ½ tsp every 4 hours
9-9.9	65	1.5	100	1 ½ tsp every 4 hours
10-10.9	70	2	130	2 tsp every 6 hours
11-11.9	75	2	130	2 tsp every 6 hours
12-12.9	90	2	130	2 tsp every 4 hours
13-14	95	2.5	162	2 ½ tsp every 4 hours

Source: Adapted by Dr. Woodson from the product circular for Lortab® and Hycodan®. Safety and effectiveness in the pediatric population below the age of two years have not been established.

Hydrocodone Dosing guidelines for flu symptoms in adults		
Concentration: Hydrocodone 1 mg/tsp		
Symptom	Dose	Frequency
Cough	1 or 2 tsp	
Headache	1 or 2 tsp	
Muscle aches and pain	1 or 2 tsp	Every 4 to 6 hours as needed
Abdominal cramps	1 tsp	
Diarrhea	1 tsp	

Promethazine

Indications and usage

Promethazine, either orally or by suppository, is useful for:

- Perennial and seasonal allergic rhinitis
- Vasomotor rhinitis
- Allergic conjunctivitis due to inhalant allergens and foods

- Mild, uncomplicated allergic skin manifestations of urticaria and angioedema
- Amelioration of allergic reactions to blood or plasma
- Dermographism
- Anaphylactic reactions, as adjunctive therapy to epinephrine and other standard measures, after the acute manifestations are controlled
- Preoperative, postoperative, or obstetric sedation
- Prevention and control of nausea and vomiting associated with certain types of anesthesia and surgery
- Therapy adjunctive to meperidine or other opioid analgesic analgesics for control of post-operative pain
- Sedation in children and adults, as well as relief of apprehension and production of light sleep from which the patient can be easily aroused
- Active and prophylactic treatment of motion sickness
- Antiemetic therapy in postoperative patients.

Warnings from the promethazine product circular
"Promethazine should not be used in pediatric patients less than two years of age because of the potential for fatal respiratory depression.

Postmarketing cases of respiratory depression, including fatalities, have been reported with use of promethazine in pediatric patients less than two years of age. A wide range of weight-based doses of promethazine has resulted in respiratory depression in these patients.

Caution should be exercised when administering promethazine to pediatric patients two years of age and older. It is recommended that the lowest effective dose of promethazine be used in pediatric patients two years of age and older and concomitant administration of other drugs with respiratory depressant effects be avoided."

Homemade Promethazine Oral Suspension

Formula

- 125 cc clean water
- 1 tbsp sugar
- 1 tbsp grain alcohol (15 cc of 95% ethanol)
- ¼ tsp flavoring
- Promethazine 25 mg tablets # 12.5 (twelve and one half 25 mg tablets)

Recipe

Mix the water, sugar, ethanol and favoring and stir. Add the promethazine tablets and give them time to dissolve. Use a blunt end of an unsharpened pencil to crush any remaining fragments. Tighten the lid and shake well. Write the date formulated, contents, concentration, and instructions on the container label and store in a cool, dry and dark place.

Suggested label

- Promethazine Elixir: 12.5 mg promethazine per tsp
- DANGER KEEP OUT OF REACH OF CHILDREN
- Shake well before using. Store in a cool, dry, dark place.

- Date formulated: _____
- Compounded by: _____

Children's dose

See table: *Promethazine dosing in children*

Adult dose

½ up to 2 tsp by mouth every 4 to 6 hours as needed for nausea, abdominal cramps, or nasal congestion

Promethazine Oral Suspension dosing in children			
Concentration: Promethazine 12.5 mg/ tsp			
Lbs	Kg	Promethazine dose in mg	Maximum dose every 4 to 6 hours
15	7	6.25	1/2 tsp
21	10	9.37	3/4 tsp
27	12	12.5	1 tsp
33	15	18.75	1.5 tsp
39	18	18.75	1.5 tsp
45	20	25	2 tsp
51	23	25	2 tsp
57	26	25	2 tsp
63	29	25	2 tsp
69	31	25	2 tsp
75	34	25	2 tsp
81	37	25	2 tsp
Source: Dr. Woodson devised this table from the product circular Not for use in children under age 2			

Diphenhydramine

Diphenhydramine is sold by Wyeth Pharmaceuticals as Benadryl®. This drug has 101 uses. It may cause your nose and throat to feel "dried out", a condition that may be fine if taken for a runny nose but not so fine if taken for abdominal cramps. Diphenhydramine has strong antihistamine and anticholenergic effects, meaning that it blocks the parasympathetic nervous system. This nervous system is responsible for producing saliva, nasal fluid, bowel motility, contraction of the pupils, and slowing of the heart rate, among other bodily states. Therefore, this drug may reduce nasal discharge and saliva flow, slow intestinal motility to the point of causing constipation, dilate the pupils, speed the heart rate, and cause sedation.

Homemade Children's Antihistamine Suspension

Formula

- 1 cup of clean water (250 cc of clean water)
- Diphenhydramine 25 mg capsules #12.5 (Twelve and one half 25 mg diphenhydramine capsules = 312.5 mg)
- 2 tbsp sugar
- 2 tbsp grain alcohol (30 cc of 95% ethanol)
- ½ tsp of flavor

Recipe

Mix the water, sugar, ethanol, and flavoring in a lightproof container with a good lid. Add the diphenhydramine tablets and give them time to dissolve. Use a blunt end of an unsharpened pencil to crush any remaining fragments. Tighten the lid and shake well. Label the container and store in a cool, dry, and dark place.

Suggested label

- Homemade Children's Antihistamine Suspension
- DANGER KEEP OUT OF REACH OF CHILDREN

- Concentration: diphenhydramine 6.25 mg per tsp
- Date formulated: _____;
- Compounded by: _____

Children's Dose

See chart: *Diphenhydramine dose guideline for children*

Diphenhydramine dose guideline for children			
Concentration: diphenhydramine 6.25 mg/tsp			
Age	Dose in mg	Dosing	Frequency
0	6.25	1 tsp	Every 6 hours
1	6.25	1 tsp	Every 6 hours
2	6.25	1 tsp	Every 4 hours
3	6.25	1 tsp	Every 4 hours
4	6.25	1 tsp	Every 6 hours
5	6.25	1 tsp	Every 6 hours
6	12.5	2 tsp	Every 4 hours
7	12.5	2 tsp	Every 4 hours
8	12.5	2 tsp	Every 4 hours
9	12.5	2 tsp	Every 6 hours
10	12.5	2 tsp	Every 6 hours
11	12.5	2 tsp	Every 6 hours
12	12.5	2 tsp	Every 4 hours

Probenecid

Indications and usage

1) Probenecid is used in the treatment of chronic gout or gouty arthritis. 2) Probenecid is also used to prevent or treat other medical problems that may occur in the presence of too much uric acid.

Off-FDA label alternative use

Probenecid is sometimes used with certain kinds of antibiotics to make them more effective in the treatment of infections.

Homemade Probenecid Suspension for Children

Formula

- 1 cup of clean water (250 cc of clean water)
- Probenecid 500mg tablets #20 (Twenty 500 mg probenecid tablets = 10,000 mg)
- 2 tbsp sugar
- 2 tbsp grain alcohol (30 cc of 95% ethanol)
- ½ tsp of flavor

Recipe

Mix the water, sugar, ethanol, and favoring and stir. Add the probenecid tablets and give them time to dissolve. Use a blunt end of an unsharpened pencil to crush any remaining fragments. Tighten the lid and shake well. Write the date formulated, contents, concentration, and instructions on the container label and store in a cool, dry and dark place.

Suggested label

- Homemade Probenecid Suspension for Children
- Concentration: Probenecid 200 mg per tsp
- KEEP OUT OF REACH OF CHILDREN
- Date formulated: _____
- Compounded by: _____

Children's Dose

See chart: *Homemade Probenecid Suspension for Children*

Homemade Probenecid Suspension for Children				
Concentration: probenecid 200 mg/tsp				
Lb	Kg	Probenecid dose in mg	Dose guideline	Dose Frequency
15	7	100	½ tsp	2 x daily with Tamiflu
21	10	150	¾ tsp	2 x daily with Tamiflu
27	12	200	1 tsp	2 x daily with Tamiflu
33	15	200	1 tsp	2 x daily with Tamiflu
39	18	250	1 ¼ tsp	2 x daily with Tamiflu
45	20	300	1 ½ tsp	2 x daily with Tamiflu
51	23	350	1 ¾ tsp	2 x daily with Tamiflu
57	26	400	2 tsp	2 x daily with Tamiflu
63	29	500	2 ½ tsp	2 x daily with Tamiflu
Source: Dr. Woodson, published literature				

Diazepam

Diazepam is the generic name for Valium®. Valium is effective for many conditions and has a favorable safety profile. Common uses for diazepam include treatment of anxiety, insomnia, muscle aches and pains, muscle spasm, and alcohol withdrawal syndrome. Although diazepam is addictive, you can avoid that complication by keeping its use to only a few days in a row. Overdose with diazepam is not a serious concern for most people. However, because it suppresses the respiratory drive of some people, it is not recommended for those with emphysema or chronic bronchitis. Also, patients with cirrhosis should avoid the drug, which is metabolized in the liver, because a single dose will last, and last, and last.

Recommended indications and dosage of diazepam in adults and children	
ADULTS:	**USUAL DAILY DOSE**
Management of Anxiety Disorders and Relief of Symptoms of Anxiety.	Depending upon severity of symptoms--2 mg to 10 mg, 2 to 4 times daily
Symptomatic Relief in Acute Alcohol Withdrawal.	10 mg, 3 or 4 times during the first 24 hours, reducing to 5 mg, 3 or 4 times daily as needed
Adjunctively for Relief of Skeletal Muscle Spasm.	2 mg to 10 mg, 3 or 4 times daily
Adjunctively in Convulsive Disorders.	2 mg to 10 mg, 2 to 4 times daily
Geriatric Patients, or in the presence of debilitating disease.	2 mg to 2 $^1/_2$ mg, 1 or 2 times daily initially; increase gradually as needed and tolerated
PEDIATRIC PATIENTS:	
Because of varied responses to CNS-acting drugs, initiate therapy with lowest dose and increase as required.	1 mg to 2 $^1/_2$ mg, 3 or 4 times daily initially; increase gradually as needed and tolerated
Not for use in pediatric patients under 6 months. Source: Roche: Valium® product circular	

Indication and usage

1) Diazepam is indicated for the management of anxiety disorders or for the short-term relief of the symptoms of anxiety.

2) In acute alcohol withdrawal, diazepam may be useful in the symptomatic relief of acute agitation, tremor, impending or acute delirium tremens, and hallucinosis.

3) Diazepam is helpful as an adjunct for the relief of skeletal muscle spasm due to localized reflex spasm (such as inflammation of the muscles or joints, or secondary to trauma); spasticity caused by upper motor neuron disorders (such as cerebral palsy and paraplegia); athetosis; and stiff-man syndrome.

Homemade Children's Oral Sedative Suspension

Formula

250 cc clean water

2 tbsp sugar

2 tbsp grain alcohol (15 cc of 95% ethanol)

½ tsp flavoring

Diazepam 5 mg # 10 (Ten 5 mg diazepam tablets = 50 mg)

Recipe

Mix the water, sugar, ethanol, and flavoring and stir. Add the diazepam tablets and give them time to dissolve. Use a blunt end of an unsharpened pencil to crush any remaining fragments. Tighten the lid and shake well. Write the date formulated, contents, concentration, and instructions on the container label and store in a cool, dry and dark place.

Suggested label

- Diazepam Elixir: 1 mg per tsp
- DANGER KEEP OUT OF REACH OF CHILDREN
- Shake well before using. Store in a cool, dry, dark place.
- Date formulated: _____
- Compounded by: _____

Children's dose

see: *Recommended indications and dosage of diazepam in adults and children*

Azithromycin

Azithromycin is an antibiotic sold by Pfizer under the brand names Zithromax and Z-Pak. The patent for this drug expired in November 2005 so it is now available in a generic version that works equally well but is significantly less expensive. Azithromycin has very few side effects and is well tolerated by most people. It is a particularly good choice to have on hand during an influenza pandemic because its spectrum of activity is ideal for the respiratory infections that complicate influenza, including pneumonia, sinusitis, and bronchitis.

Indication and usage

Adults: Recommended Dose/Duration of Therapy[90]

- Community-acquired pneumonia (mild severity), Pharyngitis/tonsillitis (second line therapy), Skin/skin structure (uncomplicated) 500 mg as a single dose on Day 1, followed by 250 mg once daily on Days 2 through 5. Azithromycin tablets can be taken with or without food.
- Acute bacterial exacerbations of chronic obstructive pulmonary disease (mild to moderate) 500 mg QD x 3 days OR 500 mg as a single dose on Day 1, followed by 250 mg once daily on Days 2 through 5.
- Acute bacterial sinusitis 500 mg QD x 3 days
- Genital ulcer disease (chancroid) One single 1-gram dose
- Non-gonococcal urethritis and cervicitis: One single 1-gram dose
- Gonococcal urethritis and cervicitis One single 2-gram dose

Adult dosing guideline for azithromycin antibiotic tablets		
Indication	Dose	How to take it
Pneumonia	250 mg tablet	Take two tablets on the first day, then one daily for 4 additional days, then stop
Pharyngitis/tonsillitis (Throat infection)	250 mg tablet	Take two tablets on the first day, then one daily for 4 additional days then stop
Otitis Media (Ear infection)	250 mg tablet	Take two tablets on the first day, then one daily for 4 additional days, then stop
Cellulitis (Skin infection)	250 mg tablet	Take two tablets on the first day, then one daily for 4 additional days, then stop
Sinusitis (Sinus infection)	250 mg tablet	Take two tablets daily for three days, then stop.
Acute or chronic bronchitis	250 mg tablet	Take two tablets daily for three days, then stop.
Gonorrhea	250 mg tablet	8 tablets taken once as a single dose, then stop
Source: Azithromycin product circular		

Pediatric Patients: Recommended Dose/Duration of Therapy[90]

Note: Although I provide this recipe for making a homemade oral suspension from tablets, you should be aware that pre-made oral suspensions also are available commercially.

Azithromycin for oral suspension can be taken with or without food.

- Acute Otitis Media: The recommended dose of azithromycin for oral suspension for the treatment of pediatric patients with acute otitis media is 30 mg/kg given as a single dose or 10 mg/kg once daily for 3 days or 10 mg/kg as a single dose on the first day followed by 5 mg/kg/day on Days 2 through 5.
- Acute Bacterial Sinusitis: The recommended dose of azithromycin for oral suspension for the treatment of pediatric patients with acute bacterial sinusitis is 10 mg/kg once daily for 3 days.
- Community-Acquired Pneumonia: The recommended

dose of azithromycin for oral suspension for the treatment of pediatric patients with community-acquired pneumonia is 10 mg/kg as a single dose on the first day followed by 5 mg/kg on Days 2 through 5.

Homemade Azithromycin Oral Suspension

Formula

- 125 cc clean water
- 1 tbsp sugar
- 1 tbsp grain alcohol (15 cc of 95% ethanol)
- 1/4 tsp flavoring
- Azithromycin 250 mg tablets # 12.5 tablets (twelve 250 mg azithromycin tablets)

Recipe

Mix the water, sugar, ethanol, and flavoring and stir. Add the azithromycin tablets and give them time to dissolve. Use a blunt end of an unsharpened pencil to crush any remaining fragments. Tighten the lid and shake well. Write the date formulated, contents, concentration, and instructions on the container label and store in a cool, dry, and dark place.

Suggested label

- Azithromycin Suspension 125 mg per tsp
- KEEP OUT OF REACH OF CHILDREN
- Shake well before using. Store in a cool, dry, dark place.

- Date formulated: _____
- Compounded by: _____

Children's dose

See: *Dosing guide for homemade azithromycin oral suspension in children*

Dosing guide for homemade azithromycin oral suspension in children			
Concentration azithromycin = 125 mg/tsp			
Lbs	Kg	Dose of Azithromycin Oral Suspension	Dose in tsp given once daily for 5 days
15-20	7-9	62.5	½ tsp
21-26	10-12	94	¾ tsp
27-32	12-14	125	1 tsp
33-38	15-17	156	1 ¼ tsp
39-45	18-19	185	1 ½ tsp
45-50	20-22	185	1 ½ tsp
51-56	23-25	250	2 tsp
57-62	26-28	250	2 tsp
63-68	29-30	281	2 ¼ tsp
69-74	31-33	281	2 ½ tsp
75-80	34-36	375	3 tsp
81-90	37-40	375	3 tsp
90+	40+	Use Adult guidelines	

Chapter 10

PANDEMIC PSYCHOLOGY

If the Great Bird Flu Pandemic is severe, we will find ourselves living in a challenging time. Simply put, the psychological response to a pandemic event falls into one of three phases: (1) The ante-pandemic phase of accepting the possibility that a pandemic is coming, (2) the pandemic phase of living through trauma from the event, and (3) the pandemic aftermath that will include the loss of loved ones and a changed world. Effective coping at each phase requires different skills. Having insight into how these major life events may affect people is the first step in coping.

Mental resilience

Psychological resilience is an attribute that will make dealing with the life-altering events of a pandemic more manageable. Resilience, the ability to bounce back, to come to terms with changed circumstances, and to carry on, is a trait that we can learn. Major distress, pain, sadness, and anxiety cannot be avoided, but they can be handled. We can adopt viewpoints, ask questions, and take actions, which will guide us in helping each other and ourselves. The American Psychological Association has produced an informative brochure on this subject, which is reproduced as a Resource on the BFM website. [91]

The psychological stress of loss and trauma

The most serious potential loss a person can experience during the pandemic is the death of a spouse, child, or parent. Next comes loss of a job, wealth, or prestige. These losses are the fuel for a well-understood psychological process, leading most commonly to *depression, anxiety, and posttraumatic stress disorder.*

These losses are among the most significant that anyone can experience, and, unfortunately, all are likely to occur during a severe pandemic. Losses of this type play a major role in the development of depression, anxiety, and posttraumatic stress disorder. Physical injury or threat of violence as a result of civil disorder or lawlessness--especially in association with the crimes of assault, murder, and rape--also commonly induce these psychological states.

The grieving process

The predictable sequence during grieving is numbness, denial, anger, despondence, depression, and hopefully, resolution through acceptance. In a healthy response to loss, the final phase of the grief process is accompanied by the emergence of a new emotional structure that is deeper and more integrated than prior to the loss. Failure to make a healthy adjustment to loss often leads to the development of unhealthy mental states and even suicide in some cases.

No one will remain untouched by this emergency if it is severe. With no easy, psychological solutions to these problems, treatment could be complicated by the lack of access to professional psychiatric care and medications. Those suffering from unhealthy mental conditions will need the help of their family and friends.

Signs and symptoms caused by loss or trauma

As in other branches of medicine, a *sign in psychiatry* is something that you observe in another person. In the psychiatric context, *symptoms* are dysfunctional feelings or thoughts the person has about the self, others, or life in general.

Signs of depression

Withdrawal from other people, both emotionally and physically, is a common sign of depression. People suffering with this condition may appear less well groomed than usual, and their standards of personal hygiene can drop. They look sad and dispirited. Depression can cause people to be hypersensitive to comments made during routine conversation, appearing as inappropriate behavior such as an angry outburst, crying, or nervousness. Depression makes it hard for people to work or think, and if they are forced to work, they can exhibit physical symptoms that prevent them from that activity. Their sleeping patterns can be disrupted, or they may want to sleep more than usual. Their eating patterns may change, and they can gain or lose significant amounts of weight. They don't seem to care about things they once deemed important. They appear to have given up and quit trying.

Symptoms of depression

Sadness and loss of an interest in things that a person used to enjoy are cardinal feelings with depression. The patient may feel remote from others, isolated, and alone. Guilt is a common theme as is feeling worthless and "good for nothing". The depressed often carry on an incessant conversation in their minds, criticizing faults and weaknesses. This unhealthy mind state is known as *rumination.* They feel worthless, unloved, and unlovable. They have lost hope for redemption or forgiveness for the things about which they feel guilty. They also may experience *survivor's guilt,* questioning why they are alive while their loved ones died. Some people may contemplate suicide. They feel empty inside. Some are tortured by the feeling of a great emptiness within their chest. Its like their heart has been replaced with giant hole. They may think that others are talking about them and even planning to harm them. They feel unacceptable and unloved.

Signs of anxiety

Nervousness is the hallmark of simple anxiety. The nervous person seems unsettled and uncomfortable in most situations. They may seem restless, agitated, and fidgety, having trouble staying still.

A special type of anxiety is a panic attack. One minute everything is fine with a person, while the next brings on uncomfortable behavior. Although most panic attacks are unassociated with hyperventilation, some are. Hyperventilation means breathing too deeply or rapidly for the needs of the body, leading to fainting or other physical symptoms. A person undergoing a panic attack may have a rapid heart rate and excessive perspiration. These *panic attacks* are associated with *hyperventilation syndrome.*

Symptoms of anxiety

Symptoms of anxiety include feeling nervous and unsettled inside. The person feels that something is not right but is unable to say what is wrong. He may have difficulty sleeping, awaking in the morning more tired and sore than he went to bed. Back and shoulder pain are common as is tension in the neck. Eating can increase or decrease, with weight gain or loss, respectively. Some people suffer chest or abdominal pains that mimic serious medical disorders. A common presentation is the sensation of tightness around the neck, or in the throat, especially anteriorly near the larynx.

In addition to hyperventilation, other symptoms may accompany the panic attack, including nausea, air hunger, headache, chest pains, dizziness, an inability to concentrate or think clearly, and, in some cases, fainting. This disorder is more unpleasant than dangerous, although the person experiencing it often thinks she is dying. Placing a paper bag or plastic baggie over the mouth and nose and slowly rebreathing the exhaled air helps restore lost balance between blood acid and alkali, and it will help relieve the symptoms.

Signs of post-traumatic stress disorder

Post-traumatic stress disorder (PTSD) occurs more commonly in women than men. In women, sexual or physical abuse is its most common cause. In men, PTSD is often triggered by involvement in violent, life-threatening situations and experience of trauma during wartime. The deaths and civil disorder that could occur during a pandemic will certainly provide a fertile ground for the emergence of this disorder. People with PTSD can become withdrawn but also argumentative. PTSD caused many of the cases of "battle fatigue" observed during past wars. They often exhibit behavior similar to those with depression or anxiety. To relieve the stress, pain, and tension associated with this condition, they commonly self-medicate with alcohol and drugs. Some people with PTSD have angry outbursts that can become violent. Irrational behavior and aggressive sexual acting are other features in patients with PTSD.

Symptoms of post-traumatic stress disorder

In addition to sharing similar elements with both depression and anxiety, the symptoms of PTSD include the distinguishing characteristic of *flashback*, or the reliving of the traumatic event with dream-like clarity. People with PTSD feel alienated and cut off from their family and friends. They feel sullen, have lost hope for a better future, and can become very cynical.

Temporary psychiatric care

If access to professional psychiatric help is available, the person suffering from these disorders should be encouraged to consult them. During a time of crisis when access to professional help and medications for treatment of these disorders is unavailable, the strategy recommended by organizations like the American Red Cross is to help the person cope with the direct consequences of the events without trying to delve deeply into their meaning or long-term consequences. The objective is to help the person remain functional rather than become another casualty during the emergency when resources are stretched to the limit. I have adapted and modified this approach for the Bird Flu Manual by suggesting we use the mind's natural methods of dealing with the issues of depression, anxiety, and PTSD as an acceptable temporary approach. These naturally occurring states include suppression, denial, and regression.

Dealing with harmful thoughts and feelings during the emergency

It is important to recognize when a member of your family or a friend is displaying any of the signs and symptoms suggestive of these mental disorders. The sooner positive steps are taken to deal with the condition, the better. Because you may be stressed already in coping with your own survival, a mental breakdown of a loved one, friend, or neighbor can become advanced before you or others notice. Remember, the objective is to help the person return to a reasonable level of functioning and avoid complete emotional collapse.

Suppression of traumatic memories as an aid to a return to function

A natural way many people manage severe trauma is to suppress painful memories. This measure is very effective in helping people regain their footing and return to a functional level. Suppressing unpleasant memories is a form of active forgetting, as in changing the mental channel whenever painful thoughts arise. This active forgetting prevents people from becoming too absorbed in their misery. Thinking harmful thoughts repeatedly is a habit with bad consequences. While some traditional psychotherapeutic approaches encourage the patient to experience their pain, and even in some cases to relive the traumatic events that caused the damage, this approach is to be avoided during the emergency. Rather the person suffering this type of injury should put these thoughts and feelings aside and move on. In contrast to modern psychotherapy, first aid for these major psychological traumas during an emergency concentrates on helping the victim suppress the memory of traumatic events. The person is encouraged to devote themselves to one or more tasks that absorb their time and energy. The objective is to forget the events and refrain from dwelling on them.

Denial is the last defense of the ego

Another natural way the mind has to deal with traumatic loss is denial. This mind tool allows us to pretend that everything is fine. Like an actor playing a part, the more we can let ourselves adopt this attitude, the better we feel. Denial is a powerful psychological defense mechanism that has evolved in humans over the millennia. That it remains universally throughout humankind is a testament to its survival advantage. Denial is an important and useful technique for humans to weather tough times and keep going forward despite great loss and suffering. Denial, enhanced by the active suppression of traumatic memories or thoughts, is a powerful combined tool for combating mental collapse during an emergency.

To help someone maintain denial, avoid discussing the facts of the person's loss unless he brings it up. In that case, listen to what the person has to say rather than trying to force him to "face reality." Completely avoid this tactic. Making a suffering person see the reality of her plight is not the objective here. Being supportive and encouraging is. Things usually have a way of working out in the end, and many times even for the best although that likelihood seems improbable at the time. Painting as optimistic a view as possible is the best approach.

Regression is the refuge of the psychiatrically injured

A mental and behavioral change likely to be prevalent during a severe influenza pandemic is regression among those who have experienced major losses or trauma. This response is another common and natural method our minds have of dealing with these conditions. While people living with and around the person experiencing regression may be disconcerted by the change in the person's behavior, their strategy should avoid trying to bring the person out of the state and instead tolerate and support the person. Given the circumstances, trying to force the person to return to a prior level of maturity could result in total emotional collapse. The regressed state may be the highest attainable at the moment. As the person begins to recover, she will naturally regain her equilibrium and begin exhibiting more mature behavior. In the meantime, a good strategy is to accept and support the person. She will return to normal in her own time, when she is able.

The use of unconventional approaches during the emergency

Recommending the use of memory suppression, denial, and tolerance of regressed states will sound like heresy to many psychological professionals who have labored long to help patients uproot these behaviors sometimes perceived as barriers to recovery. Admittedly, these alternative methods have limited value and are far from ideal. They are poor alternatives to modern psychiatric treatments, and I suggest them here only for use in the event that access to professional psychiatric help and therapy is unavailable. Furthermore, I suggest them based on the mind's natural way of dealing with crisis.

Supportive Group discussion

A regular gathering each evening to discuss the day's events, problems, and rumors is a good idea for neighborhoods in the time of pandemic. Meetings such as this can serve several important purposes, among the foremost is a way to establish and increase cohesion of those undergoing the pandemic.

Serious psychiatric problems

Serious psychological and psychiatric problems require professional treatment. If during or after the pandemic someone becomes ill with a sever mental disorder, the best advise is to get them into the care of a professional therapist or psychiatric facility for treatment. The unconventional suggestions provided in this manual should be regarded as first aid only. They are suggested as a means of helping prevent the person experiencing mental trauma from having a total breakdown. They may or may not help. At most, these methods should be viewed as a band-aid, not treatment. They are intended for temporary use only until a mental health professional can evaluate and treat the patient properly.

Remaining sane during the pandemic

Am I going nuts?

While stress and change will affect everyone during a pandemic, most people will manage to carry on without being at risk of mental collapse. In the population as a whole, during times of great stress, one in five people are at risk for suffering a breakdown with one in ten likely to have this reaction. Two people can be subjected to a severe tragedy of a similar nature with one suffering a breakdown and the other managing to cope. Nevertheless, stress is stress, and it can make life unpleasant. Feeling sad, anxious, and hopeless in response to severe loss and trauma is normal. It does not necessarily mean you are developing one of the psychiatric problems described above. These normal feelings become disorders only when they totally dominate a person and make it hard or impossible for that person to carry out regular activities. So don't assume you have a problem if you share some of the feelings typically associated with depression, anxiety or PTSD. In fact, if you don't experience some of these feelings after a loss or trauma, this state is abnormal. These symptoms become disorders only when they distort a person's view of himself and his world in irrational ways.

Staying sane in an insane world

A severe pandemic could cause a large number of people to become suddenly and involuntarily unemployed. Schools may close, and it may become difficult, if not impossible, for most people to enjoy the freedoms and privileges they took for granted ante-pandemic. Worst of all, the TV might not work! Whatever will we do with ourselves?

Many people will find it difficult to adjust to the changed circumstances of an emergency. Life will be different than before, more physically and mentally demanding. Each day, people will spend more time just satisfying the basic needs of their family and friends. While this work is important, it will not be what people are used to, and it will be hard because new skills are needed to carry it out. Much of the work will be more physically strenuous than people in the developed world are accustomed.

Plan to develop innovative ways to entertain your family. Policies like social distancing or quarantines may limit our activities, requiring us to remain at home most of the time. In the event we loose electric power, with no TV or radio as a diversion, it will be necessary for us to draw upon our creativity to discover productive and entertaining activities.

Reading is fundamental

Reading books will be an important pastime for many people, and particularly for all school-age children and adolescents. Throughout history, children have received their educations by reading books. Virtually all subjects except mathematics can be taught in this way. The classic Greeks as well as the Romans relied on an educational plan led by a tutor, who assigned students a reading lesson. After the reading, the tutor and the child then discussed the work.

The games children play

Children need to play, but depending on their ages, they also need supervision. In families that have experienced pandemic-related trauma, a child may express semi- and unconscious emotions and thoughts during play that they are unable to express consciously. An observant yet unobtrusive adult should be alert to the play of small children, monitoring their banter and behavior for themes. During play therapy, an adult may help a child express pent-up feelings at a time when the child feels safe to express feelings that seem like "make-believe."

Gardening for mental and physical health

Many adults already enjoy gardening. The pandemic period is likely to last between 12 and 18 months giving you plenty of time to grow fruits and vegetables. Even after the pandemic, stores will take time to reopen and restock with fresh fruits and vegetables. In most areas, gardeners can substitute store-bought produce with a large variety of fresh fruits and vegetables. Those with a green thumb will have an advantage, but even those with little or no experience can learn by beginning with a few basic books on gardening techniques.[92] <u>Books</u>

Maintain as normal a life pattern as possible

An important way for families and individuals to ward off negative psychological effects of the pandemic will be to maintain as much normality in their lives as possible. Patterns should follow a normal routine--going to bed in the evening, waking early, eating at meal times, and maintaining standards of home and personal hygiene. Letting these things slip will send you and your family down a degenerative slope and reinforce negative mind states like depression, anxiety, and anger. Maintaining standards of behavior, dress, and conduct is reassuring at a deep level. These standards are familiar and expected, and in return, everyone knows how to behave and react. This removes uncertainly about the immediate situation, helping to reduce stress as well as other negative emotions.

Survival of the fittest

Adults will be responsible for many activities to keep their families fed, housed, clothed, and warm during a severe pandemic period. As discussed, the work will be different than what most people performed before the pandemic, and some of these tasks, while simple, will require greater effort because of unfamiliarity and the usual inactivity of most people living in advanced societies. Physically fit people will have of the advantage of surviving the challenge of pandemic.

The only constant is change

If we are destined to live through a severe influenza pandemic, this time will be unlike anything most people have ever experienced. The pandemic will end one day, and when it does, things will return to normal. However, during the pandemic, the return to normality may seem always a long way in the future. This is a delusion, not truth.

An experience as dramatic as a major influenza pandemic most certainly will affect everyone. In the end, we will adapt to the world anew. Some people may be traumatized so severely that they will require many years to come to terms with the change. Some may never do so. However, most will adapt, recovering fully. Bad memories will fade, to be replaced by new wounds. The old adage holds true, even in dealing with pandemic: time heals all wounds.

CHAPTER 11:

Part III: Home Preparedness
Pandemic Survival Plan

The advent of a severe influenza pandemic will be a survival challenge for everyone. No one will escape the threat irrespective of wealth, rank, or intelligence. Pandemic influenza will not discriminate based on race, creed, or national origin. We will all be thrust into the same caldron, from which the virus and our struggle with it will cast our fate. <u>Pandemic Survival Plans</u>

Write down your plan

Your first priority should be writing a pandemic survival plan. A good plan is one that includes where your family will live during the pandemic, with whom you will partner, and how you will provide for your family's basic needs. Draft this plan as soon as you accept that risk from an influenza pandemic is real and high. When deciding about how much time, effort, and money to commit to pandemic preparedness, consider that your goal is to survive the duration of the pandemic. To insure this survival requires having an appreciation of how the pandemic could affect your family and way of life. With this appreciation comes a better idea of what needs to be prepared and how you can meet basic challenges such as adequate supplies of food, water, and electrical power. <u>General Preparedness</u>, <u>Books</u>, & <u>Water</u>

Surviving well during the pandemic doesn't require a permanent or even the best solution, only a solution that is "good enough." Purchase a composition notebook and keep it with you while you read this section of the manual. As you go along, write down thoughts and ideas in your notebook so that you remember them when you prepare your PSP. In this way, you'll have a head start on the plan.

Pandemic Survival Plan triggers

Triggers are milestones in the evolution of the pandemic influenza virus that cause you to take certain predetermined actions. Triggers are an important way to help one objectively, logically, and comprehensively initiate certain steps in a PSP at an appropriate time. In times of great stress and risk, you want to be prepared rather than flying by the seat of your pants. Preparing for a severe influenza pandemic is time-consuming and expensive. And you want to avoid implementing your plan if it is unnecessary. The trigger schema presented here is an example of a template for your own tailored plan that will reflect the unique character and priorities suited to your situation.

As discussed earlier, the H5N1 bird flu has acquired all the genetic characteristics it needs to establish pandemic status except one. When and if it will take this last evolutionary step is unknown. However, the factors I've elucidated point to a high likelihood of this occurrence. As time passes, the risk increases that the pandemic will unfold. Careful planning is the hallmark of sound preparation, and a good plan will include a list of items to have on hand. It also will cover how to make the best use of time and available resources as well as establish a logical point at which these items should be obtained. The plan should pinpoint the appropriate time to take certain actions based on the state of the pandemic. If people wait too long to create or implement their plans, the items they need may no longer be available or cost too much. On the other hand, people also should refrain from jumping prematurely and buying supplies that they will not need.

Having a pre-determined PSP trigger for each important action specified in the plan provides discipline. If "X" happens, it is time to implement "Y". Following this approach will reduce the tendency for people to be uncertain of when to act. No discussion or decision will be needed when the triggers are clearly defined.

As the virus progresses along its evolutionary path, more and more people will begin to perceive the risk and start their preparations. If you wait too long to prepare, you could get caught without the essential supplies your family needs to survive the pandemic. Using triggers that are tied to the actual behavior of the virus to help guide the execution of your plan is a sensible solution to this problem.

In this manual, I refer often to the WHO Influenza Pandemic Phase system as a key barometer of bird flu activity. As described earlier, the WHO has been slow to advance their alert phase. Despite this shortcoming, this alert system remains the best model to follow for gauging the virus's developmental progress.

What is needed is a way to determine the *de facto* or actual WHO Phase we are in now rather than waiting for an official announcement, which may be slow in coming. The triggers we follow therefore must be governed by events on the ground, specifically the *behavior of the virus rather than the declarations of the WHO*. Part I of this manual gives you the tools and knowledge needed to help you determine the virus' progress. Armed with this information, you can make an independent assessment of the progress the virus is making on its pandemic path. A review of information presented in media reports will help you extrapolate meaning and impact. You will be able to interpret the facts yourself rather than relying only on optimistic interpretations and announcements from the news services and government agencies. I will monitor the events leading to the pandemic and maintain a "de facto" WHO Pandemic Alert Phase on the BFM website based on these principals. Since, in my opinion for the reasons detailed in Part I of this manual, we have been in de facto WHO Pandemic Alert Phase 4 since the summer of 2005, your preparation status and plan should be implemented given that degree of risk.

Your pandemic refuge

Taking refuge within the neighborhood

Most people will be better off staying in their well-prepared and provisioned home than on the crowded road, in the midst of potential fuel shortages with other pandemic refugees and the criminals seeking to prey on them. If you live in or near a high crime area, you could investigate a safer place to stay during the pandemic in light of certain rising crime rates if police services deteriorate. If relocation is impossible, discuss how you can make your neighborhood safer with family and friends.

The rural retreat

Some people may wish to locate a pandemic refuge outside the city. Remember, it is unnecessary to implement a long-lasting solution. All you need is a temporary solution that is good enough to get you through the 18-month pandemic period. The land you choose should be large enough to accommodate everyone going with you, and it needs to have the resources needed to sustain your group. <u>Books</u>

If you are an urban resident and plan to leave the city for a retreat in the country, do so early in the pandemic. If your city has the misfortune to be one of the first areas affected by the pandemic, be aware that the federal government's plan relies heavily upon the imposition of quarantines to contain the spread of the pandemic. You might find the road out of town blocked if you wait too long. At a news conference in October 2005, President Bush indicated that he was considering just such an action as quarantining American cities to prevent the spread of avian influenza.

Recommended Pandemic Survival Plan triggers

Trigger: WHO Phase 4

- Locate your pandemic refuge

- Identify the "natural" members of your Pandemic Survivor's Group.

- Make contact with key potential members of your Group and begin a serious dialog about the pandemic.

- Begin bird flu education of all potential members of your Group.

- Complete a thorough written Pandemic Survival Plan.

- Define your Spartan Energy Budget. Determine how you will meet your alternative energy needs and what items you require to do so

- Specify and identify suppliers for the items in your family's Spartan Energy Plan

- Begin purchase of all devices for your family's Spartan Energy Plan

- Determine what foods to stockpile

- Begin your food stockpile.

- Evaluate potential water sources. Devise a plan for collecting, purifying, and filtering water for home consumption.

- Purchase and install all the items necessary for your alternative water supply plan, but do not fill them with water yet.

- Begin saving cash. Try and put away enough free cash to support your family's needs for 3 months. Find the best way to purchase 1/10th oz American Eagle gold and 1 oz American Eagle silver coins. Convert some cash into these coins for use later.

- Purchase all the items listed in the manual for the Flu Treatment Kit. Discuss getting a 3-month supply of essential medications with your doctor. Ask her to look over and consider prescribing the medications listed in the FTK for you to have on hand in the event a pandemic occurs.

- Monitor the behavior of the bird flu virus and look for signs of localized human-to-human spread that signifies Phase 5 has begun. I will be announcing my view of what pandemic stage we are in on the BFM.com website.

- Consider constructing a solarium for passive home heating.

- If you plan on storing vegetables in a root cellar, dig one now while you can still rent a backhoe and buy lumber at the hardware store.

- Review your plan and look for weaknesses. If possible, try to locate supplies you overlooked or augment supplies or items you need.

Trigger: WHO Phase 5

- Complete food stockpile ASAP. Panic buying may cause some demand shortages during Phase 5, but no true supply shortages will occur until about one month after Phase 6 actually begins.

- Begin formal meetings on pandemic preparedness with the key members of your group.

- While each family needs to write their own PSP that provides for their specific needs, the PSG as a whole also needs to craft a plan that deals with issues that are applicable to the entire group rather than any specific individual. For instance, the group PSP might include items like group safety and security, mortuary preparations, the neighborhood health network and others.

- Activate your group neighborhood medical network plan. Obtain needed supplemental supplies for provision of advanced home care. All members of the medical network begin regular meetings for planning and implementation for the time when home care will predominate hospital care.

- Provide for remote group members to return to the group's refuge on a moment's notice by giving each an Emergency Travel Kit. The kit needs to be kept close by at all times. Make plans for what to do about pets of remote group members.

- Begin your home or group garden. Consider obtaining or building a temporary greenhouse or cold frame. Obtain enough tools, non-hybrid seeds, fertilizer, lime, and insecticides needed for your garden to last for 2 years without need for re-supply.

- Complete your purchase of any weapons and ammunition you plan to have on hand for home and group defense. Sales of these items are likely to become restricted after the declaration of Phase 6.

- Obtain more gasoline and LP gas for your stockpile, if needed. Consider purchasing more Spartan Energy Plan generating and storage devices (PV panels and deep cycle storage batteries) now because they will be unavailable once Phase 6 is declared. Demand will be enormous and supply will be limited by lack of adequate production facilities.

- Review your plan and look for weaknesses. If possible, try to locate supplies you overlooked or augment supplies or items you need.

Trigger: WHO Phase 6

- If the case fatality rate is < 2%, then a mild pandemic is developing.

- If the case fatality rate is >2% but less than 5% then a moderate pandemic is developing.

- If the case fatality rate is > 5% a severe pandemic is developing.

- In the event of a severe pandemic, all adults should take an emergency leave of absence from work and focus entirely on pandemic preparedness from this point forward. If the case fatality rate is less than 5% or the rate is unclear, some adults should take leave while others continue employment until the pandemic declares itself.

- Recall all remote group members to the refuge.

- College students should drop their courses and return home to help the family and group with preparations.

- Complete all preparations.

- Begin holding daily AM planning and action meetings with key Group members. Begin daily PM group meetings with the entire group to discuss the day's activities and unmet needs and concerns. Plan for these meetings to continue for the duration of the pandemic.

- Carefully monitor reports on the pandemic's progress but disregard misinformation and misguided attempts at reassurance that will only cause the unprepared to remain so. Opinions will vary widely, and so will advice. Stick to the case fatality rate of those sick with the disease. That is the information of importance. Nothing else matters. If the rate is 5% or higher, a severe pandemic has begun with the most dire consequences likely. The affects of a moderate pandemic will still be dreadful and cause significant economic and social displacement but not nearly as bad as we can expect from a severe event.

- Hold your ground and don't panic. Keep your group together and be hopeful because you are prepared.

Don't leave your prepared refuge. Your chances of survival are much better hunkered down where you are than as a refugee. Avoid becoming a refugee at all costs.

- Monitor the Internet sites like Fluwickie.com for updates. They will be providing raw unfiltered data that will require interpretation but will actually be more reliable than some official media.

- Fill your water containers.

- Review your plan and look for weaknesses. If possible, try to locate supplies you overlooked or augment supplies or items you need.

Trigger: Pandemic human bird flu reaches your country

- Stay cool. You and your group are as ready as you can be.

- Any adults who have not already done so should take an emergency leave of absence from their work to focus on completing all pandemic preparedness tasks.

- Continue group meetings everyday. The AM meetings should be reserved for the group leadership and focus on planning and plan implementation. The PM community meetings provide a venue for any group member to speak about their needs and concern. Rumors should be openly discussed and debunked. Fear and panic is best controlled in this way. Stress to each member of the group that their attendance at these PM meetings is of the utmost importance.

- Rumors are always the currency of crisis. Almost all rumors will be false. Disregard them. The quality of the information available will progressively deteriorate from this point forward. The best way to debunk a rumor is to discuss it openly, letting the light of reason burn through and destroy it.

- Above all, work to allay fears and maintain the unity of the group. Fear of the unknown will be high. Discussion will help.

- The group leadership must strive always to keep everyone together. There will be great pressure on some members of the group to leave and go somewhere else that "might be safer." That scenario is improbable and traveling will certainly be hazardous. Try to keep the group together. Having implemented a solid PSP that you and your group fulfilled is the best guarantee that your refuge will serve the needs of all your group's members better than or as well as any other location.

- Implement full self-containment procedures now, even though you have access to water and electrical service and police protection.

Trigger: Pandemic bird flu reaches your community

- This is an expected event that you have prepared for. Nothing has changed. Your group is ready to take care of itself. Do not be afraid. Remember that almost everyone will survive, even those who become ill. You are not alone. Everyone in the group is working for the benefit of all the other members giving each the best chance of survival.

Trigger: Pandemic flu affects members of your group

- Early in the pandemic, hospitals and doctor's offices should be functional. Seek conventional treatment. Since the U.S. Government predicts that 8 in 9 flu patients will be treated at home, you are prepared to provide this service.

- Begin home schooling your children if you have not already done so since the social distancing policy will be implemented soon closing the schools.

- Follow your plan. Continue the AM leadership meeting and the PM community meetings. Encourage open discussion and information exchange. Information quality and reliability will be poor even from authoritative sources reported in the media. Discuss rumors, but don't let them hold sway. Debunk them, as they will be baseless for the most part.

- Pull together and help the flu patients and families of these patients cope. Don't be concerned about getting the flu. As stated in the text, "don't worry about contacting the flu, it will contact you". There is really very little chance of avoiding exposure to the virus no matter what you do.

Trigger: The First Pandemic Wave Ends

- We can hope that the first pandemic wave will be relatively mild as was seen in the spring of 1918. Waves last 2 or 3 months. Do not fall victim to hopeful comments by many who think the pandemic is over. This is not consistent with the facts from the past. Above all, keep your group together.

- Able adults should return to work at this point if they have a job available. The inter-pandemic wave period will be the lull before the storm.

- Re-supply any depleted stocks of food, water, and alternative energy devices.

- Review your plan and look for weaknesses. Rotate food stocks and stored water. Add new supplies that you realized were needed or desirable during the first wave.

- Maintain and intensify your home gardening activities. Look for opportunities to purchase needed tools, seeds, fertilizer, and lime.

- Family finances could be in a terrible mess at this point especially if there has been widespread involuntary unemployment. Payments and bills may be overdue. If you find yourself in this condition, *conserve your remaining savings and cash.* Ignore the bill collectors. You may actually be technically bankrupt but don't worry about it now. A lot of folks are going to be in this shape, so you will not be alone. The creditors won't be able to act decisively until after the end of the pandemic. At that time, there will be tremendous pressure to accommodate debtors. The U.S. Congress is likely to pass legislation requiring creditors to reschedule debts, which will solve the problem. What you are going to need to get through this emergency is cash, and gold and silver coins to meet your everyday needs. Remember, the worst is yet to come.

- Decide whether to continue home schooling the group's children or return them to regular school. Past timing of pandemic waves supports continued home schooling. Schools are likely to be closed again before long. The effects of the first wave and the knowledge that a second more severe one is on the way are likely to be very distracting for children and teachers, making the task of providing conventional classroom instruction very difficult.

- College students should remain at the refuge because it is unlikely that they will be able to complete a semester, even if their school reopens before the second wave arrives. Home study and helping out in the community and within the group, like providing home schooling for the youngsters, will be a productive activity.

- Consider adding new members to the group who might need help or bring with them additional skills that could be of value to the group.

Trigger: The Second Pandemic wave begins

- This was the bad one in 1918 so "batten down the hatches and full speed ahead".

- All adults take an emergency leave of absence from work.

- Anyone away from the group's refuge must return ASAP.

- Keep children at home, and college students should stop attending class and begin helping with the group.

- It won't be long before civil society begins to unravel. The hospitals are likely to go first. Food shortages will become apparent.

- The crime rate will rise. If food becomes unavailable, riots will occur.

- Continue your routine--AM leadership meeting, PM community meetings.

- Begin a 24-hour neighborhood safety patrol to help guard against crime.

- Communicate with local police or sheriff contacts for guidance and for information on crime in your area.

Trigger: Closure of hospitals, clinics, and doctor's offices

- If medical resources become limited as expected, hospitals and doctor's offices will close. Medical professionals participating in your PSG will then be free to return to the neighborhood and activate the medical network. Since reliable hospital care will not be available until after the conclusion of this wave, almost all care will occur at home.

Trigger: Mortuary services become overwhelmed

- Expect the number of sick people in the area around you and within your group to rise. Mortuary services will soon be overcome and unable to accept new bodies. Temporary morgues will be established, but burial within the neighborhood of deceased group members is a better way to keep track of them than giving that responsibility to the authorities at this point in the pandemic.

Trigger: Failure of the electric grid

- In the event that this occurs, the risk for civil disorder and anarchy will be high. If you have considered this in your PSP and have a neighborhood defense plan, implement it now.

Trigger: Loss of effective community police and fire services

- The group will need to depend upon its safety officer and members of the neighborhood watch for protection usually provided by these community servants.

Deterring criminal acts and defending the group from those with violent intent will be important services to the group. Providing emergency fire service and helping group members transport sick and deceased family members will also be required of the watch.

- Monitor police scanners and local media reports for civil unrest.

- Hunker down and let the events pass by you. Don't become a refugee.

- Be prepared to defend your refuge. United you stand, divided you fall.

Trigger: End of the second wave

- What a relief!

- Have a party.

- Able-bodied adults return to work.

- Re-supply essential items. Rotate stock.

- Continue home schooling because there may be a third wave and if it comes, the schools will close again. The education your kids are getting is far superior to what organized education can do for them now. It will take years for the school system to return to the same level of the ante-pandemic. Seriously think about continuing to home school the children for a while longer.

Trigger: Beginning of the third wave

- If we have a third pandemic wave, its severity will depend on the extent of herd immunity achieved during the first two waves. If immunity is high, this wave will probably be relatively mild, if low it could be quite severe.

- Adults immune from influenza may continue working during the third wave unless they are needed at home for other critical tasks.

- Continue home schooling.

- Hospitals and clinics are likely to be open but very dysfunctional--operating at well over capacity. Acutely ill flu patients, patients who suffered complications of influenza--like stroke and heart attack, and the usual load of patients with non-influenza medical illness who have become critically ill during the many months when technically advanced healthcare and lifesaving medications were unavailable, will occupy all beds.

- College students should not yet return to class because their institutions will inevitably close again. The pandemic experience will provide a much better education than anything they could possibly have learned in school. They will experience history in the making.

- The number of group members becoming ill with bird flu during this wave will be low. Some groups might escape this wave completely. By now, the police and fire service have adjusted to the restrictions imposed upon them by the pandemic and should remain functional during the third wave. Home defense against roving gangs may still be needed but hopefully not. The crime rate, especially burglary and robbery, will skyrocket as the unemployment rate will increase and the number of economically destitute people grows--conditions historically associated with high crime rates. So, it might be wise to continue the neighborhood watch, at a lesser degree of readiness, for a year or two longer. Ask your local sheriff or police chief for guidance.

Trigger: End of the third wave.

- This will mark the end of the pandemic.

The immediate post-pandemic period

The formal ending of the pandemic will be a great relief to everyone, but coming to terms with its aftermath will present an entirely new set of seemingly endless problems. We will all be working to re-establish normal life although in truth, life will never be the same again for pandemic survivors. Nor will you ever look over your hedge at your neighbors and think of them in a disconnected, nonchalant way--not after all you went through together.

Using the post-1918 pandemic psychology as a guide, everyone will unconsciously conspire to quickly forget the pandemic and its resulting trials and tribulations. We will rush to bury the past just as fast as we rush to exhume and properly bury those who died from our group.

But don't be in too much of a rush about your dead. The morticians will have a big backlog. It is likely to take many months before they will be able to assist you. There will be a new baby boom. The economy will come back, and things will slowly return to normal. But, they won't, not completely, not for those of us who survived the Great Bird Flu Pandemic. Life will never be the same for those who survived. And when we put the world back together post-pandemic, let's do it better by relying on what we learned about people and ourselves during this crisis.

CHAPTER 12

The Pandemic Survival Group

I don't mind telling you that contemplating the onset and consequences of a severe bird flu pandemic frightens me. Figuring out the best ways for people to cope and survive in such a case has occupied much of my professional and leisure time since 2004. I am concerned that the pandemic might begin before enough people understand just how severe it could be, and before a really effective strategy for dealing with it can be established. At the federal, state, and local level the plans for coping with pandemic bird flu are likely to fail in the face of a major event. Consequently, taking a self-reliant approach to pandemic preparedness is the best way to provide your family and friends with what will be required to survive a major influenza pandemic. Pandemic Survivor Groups

People, get ready

Undoubtedly most people will provide medical care for their sick family members, friends, and neighbors within their own homes. This is contemplated in every official government plan. What will come as a surprise to many will be the need to provide critical care to severely ill people within the home setting. Organizing your family and friends in a mutually supportive group to help each other will greatly increase your odds of making it through the pandemic in one piece. You will be able to rely on this approach because you will be depending on your family, friends, and most important, upon yourself to make it work.

In a severe pandemic, you will be required to cope with the gravest medical and social consequences with virtually no outside help. Having a proper appreciation of the risks and taking prudent steps to deal with them ahead of time, are ways to cope successfully with this crisis. Since the entire country, indeed the entire world, will be affected by the pandemic, there will be no "help from outside." Essentially, there will be no unaffected "outside" to provide such help. As difficult as it may seem to accept this scenario, analysis of the impact of a major pandemic on society and its institutions indicate that most people will be forced to rely upon whatever resources they have available within their local area to sustain themselves. These resources will have to be within their home, neighborhood, and the immediate surrounding area--in other words, within walking distance of their residences.

The struggle to survive will be a strictly local affair. You will not be the only one relying on your own resources for all your basic needs. This theme will dominate the experience of virtually everyone in the United States and in the rest of the world. All people will face the same struggle to obtain basic sustenance from the local area--and all in the midst of an ongoing medical catastrophe.

Obviously, the most critical priority is to do what needs to be done to ensure the survival of your family and friends. A careful analysis of the available options existing under the conditions expected during a severe pandemic suggests that people who gather together in small- to medium-sized pandemic survivor groups can improve their chances during this emergency. The purpose of forming these groups of like-minded people is to provide mutual support and protection during the expected 18-month pandemic.

The alternative to establishing a pandemic survivor's group is to leave your home or neighborhood and become a refugee in hopes of finding better circumstances elsewhere. During my research for this manual, I found a surprisingly rich source of information within the survivalist literature. One survivalist author, who had served as a mercenary in Africa, repeatedly made the point that during a breakdown in civil order, you should above all "avoid becoming a refugee".[93] The life of a refugee is described as a living hell. Few survive unscathed, and many not at all. This survivalist resource suggests that the best way to counter civil anarchy in the wake of a crisis is "to remain on your home turf," especially if you have prepared to sustain and defend your family there. If this choice is unwise, then that author suggests identification in advance of a retreat to which you will remove yourself and family prior to the civil collapse. After considerable deliberation and research, I support his advice.

Family, friends, and neighbors

Most likely, candidates for your Pandemic Survival Group (PSG) will include your family, friends, and their family. Next are the neighbors who live around the place you will reside during the pandemic. These neighbors also will want to invite family and friends to join the PSG. This is a likely way for PSGs to naturally assemble. People gathering for mutual support and protection is nothing new. In fact, it reflects our ancient civilization. In a way, the PSG is our civilization's default organizational state, one that the pandemic will once again cause us to adopt. Ironically, our modern civilization will retreat to this regressed organizational state until life returns to normal. While it is likely that groups such as this will form wherever humans live, forming a group consciously with preparation and planning will provide the members of a PSG significant survival advantages over those who assemble haphazardly.

I can't imagine anything more important than having friends and neighbors to rely upon during this emergency. Being able to depend upon those around you for help will be a tremendous asset for every member of the PSG. A stable, prepared community lessens the likelihood that you or your family will experience problems during the pandemic. Your participation also improves the likelihood of survival for your neighbors. You may be the first to broach the subject of preparation, but by now, at least some of your neighbors are aware of the pending situation and may be considering some response.

Recruiting group members

Some of the people with whom you discuss forming a PSG will immediately see the rationale for such a gathering. However, others will judge your plan as ridiculous. Resist the urge to argue with the doubters. If bird flu continues is present evolutionary course, they will be knocking on your door soon enough. Obviously, if you live in a neighborhood or an apartment building, those who live around you, together with your friends and family, are the people you are most interested in recruiting. You might open the avenue to a discussion by giving them a copy of my first book, *The Bird Flu Preparedness Planner.*

Picking your group's first Leader

As your PSG matures, the group needs to choose a leader. The leader should be a competent planner, commander, and have the skills needed to execute the plan. Cooperation and mutual support will be essential for success. Everyone must allow the leader to lead and abide by the leader's instructions during this stressful time. Although you may not agree with all of the leader's decisions, cohesion of the group is in the interest of all its members. To help foster this cooperation, consider adopting these two rules, (1) follow the leader, and (2) stay together.

Keeping your Group together

The 18-month long pandemic will be emotionally stressful for everyone, no matter your level of preparedness. Before the pandemic actually starts, consider holding regular evening meetings with everyone in attendance. These meetings will become more frequent as the pandemic approaches and eventually will evolve into a nightly event once the pandemic begins. At these meetings, members of your community will be given an opportunity to report on progress being made in execution of the group's PSP, to ask questions or voice concerns, and to discuss and resolve any disputes or disagreements that have developed between members of the group. Discussions like this one can help prevent small disputes from erupting into fracturing events, and in fact, they may be one of the best ways to help keep your group together.

Generosity, tolerance, forgiveness, and patience are key survival virtues to cultivate among your group. Groups characterized by narcissism, paranoia, rigidity, greed, and envy will predictably self-destruct. Of course, each group's structure and form will vary according to its circumstances, a natural and healthy evolution. The groups with the best chance of survival will be those that work cooperatively to enhance the chances of survival of all their members. Sharing, sacrifice, hard work, and devotion to this goal will characterize successful groups.

When family members are scattered far and wide

The U.S. Government plans call for travel restrictions not only to the United States from pandemic-affected regions of the world but also within the states. Those family members who live far away should travel home before restrictions or quarantines are imposed. These quarantines or travel restrictions within the United States are not likely to be established until after WHO elevates the alert status to Phase 6. Prepare for this possibility by having an Emergency Travel Kit ready for each member of your family who lives far away. An Emergency Travel Kit includes an open (full-price coach round-trip) airline/train/or bus ticket home, $200 cash, a credit card, a change of clothes, toiletry items, extra medications, two water bottles, several energy bars, and essential items such as a picture ID--all stored in a small travel bag. Having such a kit ready allows your relative to grab their travel kit and make her way to the airport, train station, or bus terminal on a moment's notice. An open full-price ticket gives her a high priority on standby for the next available trip out, even without a prior reservation.

Accepting unplanned members into the group

If there is a severe pandemic, you can expect to have people totally unprepared for the emergency land on your doorstep, some with nothing more than the clothes on their back. A hallmark of civilized behavior worthy of preservation is helping those less fortunate than ourselves. In my opinion, those of us who have had the foresight to prepare for this emergency have a responsibility to have compassion for as many people as we can. Hopefully, by starting your preparations well ahead of the beginning of the pandemic, you will have an abundance of supplies to cope with the crisis. Unfortunately, those who are unprepared will pass through the most difficult portion of the pandemic under the worst of circumstances. Your kindness in reaching out to them will be rewarded by knowing you have helped as many people as possible.

Pandemic safety and security

A severe pandemic is likely to affect law enforcement officers and other first responders more than other members of the community. During a severe pandemic, police and fire personnel as well as those on the Emergency Medical Service (EMS) will be overwhelmed with calls. They may be unable to respond in a timely manner due to illness within their ranks. While everyone will come into contact with the virus eventually, police who are protecting hospitals will be repeatedly exposed to the virus.

Worst Case Scenarios

Sick people and their relatives desperately seeking treatment are likely to mob these facilities, and law enforcement personnel will have their hands full trying to keep them from over-running clinics, emergency rooms, and hospitals. The same situation will apply to firemen and EMS personnel who are responsible for transporting ill patients with flu to the hospital. The loss of these key public employees due to illness and death will place those protected by them at risk from members of society who see an opportunity to engage in crime. Without fire protection, small, otherwise easily controlled fires could quickly spread, causing major conflagrations.

Home protection measures

The group's safety officer

Your PSG should nominate a member to take responsibility for the safety and security. This person will establish a neighborhood watch for your community, which could also provide supplemental emergency fire and ambulance services for the group. In a case where law enforcement is unable to respond to a police emergency, the task of patrolling and defending the neighborhood becomes the responsibility of the safety officer.

Cooperate with security forces

During the emergency, patrolling police officers or military units are likely to pass by or even visit your neighborhood. Remember, their mission is to protect you. It is important to do all you can to cooperate completely with the police or military. Some regions of the country may be under martial law, under which civil rights are suspended and security forces have the authority to shoot on sight rioters, looters, and those breaking curfew. These forces won't distinguish between vigilantes and looters.

Make plans for group self-defense

If influenza has significantly reduced the effectiveness of your local law enforcement agency, you must consider and prepare for the possibility that your group could become the target of looters or others seeking to take advantage of the situation. Opportunists and criminals could join together in impromptu gangs in search of food, valuables, guns, and involuntary female companions. Criminals will not hesitate to exploit the vulnerable and those already weakened by illness. History is replete with accounts of raiders taking advantage of just such situations. Unfortunately, some otherwise decent people driven by despair also have been known to commit unthinkable acts during emergencies. <u>Self Defense</u>

Canine home protection

A large, well-trained family dog can be an excellent home defense choice for many people. To be effective in this role, the animal needs personal protection training by a professional. This training is widely available in many areas of the United States.

Firearms

A crucial decision that requires discussion early is whether deadly force will be used if an armed gang attacks your neighborhood. The group's safety officer needs a good grasp of state and local laws and how they apply in these situations.

The debate concerning gun rights in the United States involves the rights of individuals to possess and use firearms during times of civil order. The issue here is different because its focus is on how you can protect you family and friends during a time of civil disorder. If firearms are to be part of your group's community protection plan and you own a serviceable firearm, buy additional ammunition now for the weapon you have. If you don't have a weapon, ask your group's safety officer what additional defensive items are needed to keep your home and neighborhood safe. If your safety officer recommends a firearm, he also will be able to pinpoint an appropriate weapon type and model. Plan to spend time with someone in your group who is familiar with firearms and willing to train you on how to use one safely and effectively. Ideally, if a firearm is in your future, buy it before the pandemic begins because if you wait, the selection of guns available may be limited. Additionally, the sale of firearms and ammunition may be forbidden at some point during the pandemic by the authorities concerned about public unrest.

Vehicles and gasoline

Your group's neighborhood watch will need vehicles to respond to emergencies and calls for help. From among the inventory of vehicles available within your PSG, choose several for this purpose. Cars will be useful for patrolling the community. Having a truck will facilitate the movement of large or bulky items, sanitation, materials, and supplies through the neighborhood. You can adapt an SUV for an emergency response vehicle. Depending upon the size of your PSG and the area your group occupies, you may need one or several of these vehicles. A large PSG could outfit one SUV for neighborhood protection, one could respond to fires, and a third could serve as an ambulance and hearse. A sufficient store of gasoline must be obtained for these vehicles as well. Gasoline held in the tanks of other neighborhood vehicles could be siphoned into cans and held in reserve for use by the watch. A better solution is for the group to think ahead and purchase several 55-gallon drums suitable for gasoline. Make sure to add an appropriate quantity of fuel stabilizer to the drums when filling them. Having a rotary hand pump and hose to fill the vehicles from the large drums also will be useful. <u>Fuel Management</u>

At times during the pandemic, it could be unsafe to drive around outside of the neighborhood. Even when a semblance of civil order is present, there may be curfews. Some areas will be unsafe. Understandably, people will be curious and feel the urge to explore and find out what is going on. However, established rules should strictly limit this behavior. Those leaving the safety of the compound will be at high risk for becoming separated from the group, or worse. Their action places not only themselves at risk but also the entire group. If a gang takes hostage one of these overly curious members of your group, when placed under severe duress they are likely to reveal your group's location, details about its members, your defense preparations, and supply stockpiles.

Sanitation

Garbage pickup from communities is likely to be irregular and at times unavailable during the pandemic. This duty will default to each homeowner and PSG to solve. Allowing refuse to pile up in neighborhoods or city block is untenable. Doing so will attract rodents, packs of feral dogs, smell terrible, and be an eyesore. Each PSG needs to plan for managing garbage and implement the plan immediately upon the cessation of this vital service.

The garbage problem has many possible solutions. The most critical element of a plan to cope with trash is to have each family strictly separate biological from non-biological materials.

The members can then compost or bury these biological materials in their yard. Each household should further separate the non-biological into flammable and inflammable. Once separated, the family members could elect to burn flammable materials themselves or pass this task to the PSG members assigned to the sanitation crew. The crew would pick up these materials, burn any that are flammable, and store inflammables in a confined area until the county or private sanitation service resumes.

Don't expect usual sanitation service to resume promptly at the end of the emergency. The entire city will be crammed with mountains of refuse. Sanitation workers will be reduced in number and the local government will not have the resources available to devote more to the cleanup effort. Plan accordingly and be sure the area where you store the inflammable non-biologic refuse will be large enough to accommodate the PSG's needs for longer than expected.

Radios

Reliable information will be unavailable at the height of the crisis. If possible, obtain several sets of portable walkie-talkies for use within your group's neighborhood. Most are rated for six, seven, or even 10 miles, but they won't work over these distances when line-of-sight obstructions are present. These inexpensive radios operate reliably over approximately a one-mile radius, or even less, with trees, hills, or houses in the line-of-sight. Unlike cell phones, these devices will remain functional during the pandemic as long as you have a reliable method for charging batteries.

Better, hand-held radios that will operate over many miles are available for purchase. They cost more but may be worth having if members of your group will be traveling outside of the neighborhood during the emergency. Having these hand held units will be one of the only ways to provide your group with reliable long-range communication capability. Electronics

A police scanner might provide you with information from the police or National Guard units on patrol in the area. Setting up a ham radio base unit in the neighborhood will allow you to listen to communications between state and local emergency managers who will probably use this means of communication. A ham radio also will allow you to get news from distant places that would be difficult to come by otherwise.

Don't become a vigilante

Rest assured that after the return of law and order, people who committed major crimes during the emergency are likely to be vigorously prosecuted. Vigilante activities are crimes, and those participating in them are likely to suffer severe consequences. *Vigilantes* take the law into their own hands by deciding who is guilty of what, sentencing the person, and executing the sentence. In a country ruled by law, only the police, district attorney, judges, and juries can take these actions and then only collectively. Citizens may **not**, even in a time of civil disorder, take the law into their own hands. If they do, they have broken the law and consequently will be prosecuted for these acts once civil order is restored. In the post-pandemic environment, justice will be swift. Judges will not allow the usual motions and delays. The legal system will be pressured to move cases quickly. There will be little room in the crowded jails. Current law makes no allowances for shooting and killing someone without severe consequences, even in self-defense. So don't contemplate such actions unless you find no other options.

Crimes against persons are serious and will be prosecuted

Prosecutors may lack the resources to pursue perpetrators of *burglaries*, or property crimes where no one is injured or threatened with injury, unless item(s) stolen were of great value. *Robbery* is a theft in which the perpetrator harms or threatens to harm someone during the commission of the crime. While *assault* is a crime against a person, unless the injury is serious or committed with a gun or knife, the police will probably not pursue prosecution. However, *robbery, homicide, rape,* and *kidnapping* are likely to be pursued aggressively by law enforcement officers and district attorneys once civil order is re-established. Unfortunately, a backlog of these serious crimes may be waiting for law enforcement at the conclusion of the emergency. Law enforcement offices will remain short-staffed and under-funded for a long time after the restoration of order—an explanation for the focus on the severe felonies.

It is illegal to hold (*incarcerate*) someone against his will. Do not assume you have a right to make a "citizen's arrest." If you catch someone breaking into a home, warn them not to come back but let them go. It may endanger you to do anything further. A guard dog will be a great deterrent for this type of crime.

Mortuary preparations

Regrettably, a marked increase in deaths compressed into a short period of time is an undeniable feature of pandemic. You may have to bury a number of the dead during the pandemic. Because of the statistical phenomenon of skewing, some communities will have many more deaths than others. The most probable time for the death rate to peak will be during the most severe pandemic wave. During this peak, routine mortuary services may be unavailable due to demand, lack of electrical power, embalming supplies, caskets, and staff. Months may pass before a person who has died can be embalmed and receive a proper burial or even be issued a death certificate.

The authorities plan to set up temporary morgues in refrigerated trailers to hold the deceased. These plans work only so long as there is sufficient diesel fuel to operate the electric generators needed for the refrigeration units. The demand for these trucks will be very high and they will quickly become fully utilized. At that point or when the diesel fuel runs out, the only option will be mass burial. Inevitably there will be great confusion surrounding an event like this. The identities of many of those buried will not be known and even when they are, the location of the burial spot of a deceased family member may not be. In some locales, body pickup may become temporarily unavailable. County coroners will be reluctant to issue death certificates without proof of death. Without this, a family's options in probate court and their chances of collecting life insurance proceeds become enormously complex.

These concerns make it prudent for your group to consider burying their own dead in a temporary cemetery located within your neighborhood. Even if none of the members of your PSG dies, your group may be called on to help bury others. During the second wave of the 1918 pandemic, the death rate was higher than average among the young recruits at Camp Devens in Massachusetts, as witnessed in this letter written by a U.S. Army physician who arrived at the camp a little before the terrible second wave hit. The doctor is writing to a good friend and colleague about his first few weeks there.[94]

> *"Camp Devens is near Boston, and has about 50,000 men, or did have before this epidemic broke loose...These men start with what appears to be an ordinary attack of La Grippe or Influenza, and when brought to the hospital... It is only a matter of a few hours then until death comes (for some of them)... It is horrible. One can stand it to see one, two or twenty men die, but to see these poor devils dropping like flies sort of gets on your nerves. We have been averaging about 100 deaths per day.... It takes special trains to carry away the dead. For several days there were no coffins and the bodies piled up something fierce, we used to go down to the morgue (which is just back of my ward) and look at the boys laid out in long rows. It beats any sight they ever had in France after a battle. An extra long barracks has been vacated for the use of the morgue, and it would make any man sit up and take notice to walk down the long lines of dead soldiers all dressed and laid out in double rows".*
> -British Medical Journal, December 22, 1979

Cremation

While a funeral pyre is another option for dealing with a body, you should avoid this. The authorities may want to satisfy themselves that the person who died is indeed who you say they were, and that their manner of death was as stated. If you cremate the body, there may be inadequate remains left to make a positive identification of the deceased. Second, if the person died during an act of violence, the body will provide important evidence that the coroner and police will wish to examine carefully. Cremating a victim of a violent criminal act would impair law enforcement's ability to determine the facts of a case. Anyone who disposed of a victim of violence in this way would attract the attention of the investigators as a potential criminal suspect or co-conspirator. Burial of the body permitting exhumation and complete forensic examination of the remains would avoid these problems and be the best way to facilitate a criminal probe. In addition, cremating a body on a funeral pyre is difficult; taking a lot of valuable fuel that may be needed for cooking or heating. It is an inefficient way to dispose of the dead in the West, where most people are novices in how to prepare the body correctly for cremation. Best leave cremation to the professionals or to those cultures which have traditionally used it.

A quick burial is best

How long it takes the body to putrefy depends on the ambient temperature of its location. The warmer it is, the faster decomposition will happen. Avoid allowing the body to putrefy because a corpse in this state is more difficult to handle both from a physical and a psychological standpoint. It is in everyone's best interest to move quickly to prepare the dead and bury them quickly.

Preparing the body for burial

Those dying from influenza are no more dangerous than when they were alive. Because they do carry bacteria and viruses and might even have active bird flu virus in their secretions, routine precautions are called for—however, not more than would be the case if you were taking care of the same person with flu during life. Burial should be performed as soon as possible. Embalming the body is unnecessary since you will be burying the body quickly.

Family or friends of the deceased may wish to use a simple modification of a practice common to many ancient cultures. First, the body is undressed and laid out on a flat table. Using soap and water, the body is cleaned, dried, and wrapped in a clean cotton sheet. Tie the ends and middle of the sheet with string to keep the sheet from falling off. A coffin is unnecessary. Now the body is ready for burial and the funeral ceremony.

Transporting the dead

The same vehicle used by the neighborhood watch to transport patients to the hospital or aid station will serve well as a hearse. A natural duty for the watch will be to pick up the prepared body of the deceased and transport it to the temporary cemetery. If the body is in a decomposed state, wrap it in a plastic tarp before picking it up. Seal up the tarp and carry it in such a way as to prevent malodorous body fluids from leaking out.

Burying the dead

Most cultures and religions have specific practices that are observed before a body is buried. These rituals should be respected as far as possible. Giving the deceased funeral rites shows respect for the dead and for those who are left behind. The familiar ceremony will provide comfort, support, and closure for the family and group.

A good location for a temporary graveyard is one that is well drained, away from occupied housing, vegetable gardens, and especially from streams or wells. As the need arises, members of the watch or others within the community can dig graves. An average adult fits well in a 3 feet deep x 6 feet long x 3 feet wide grave. Once the ceremony is complete, lower the wrapped body into the bottom of the grave, cover it with 20 lbs of quick lime and fill the hole with soil. Be sure to mark the grave and keep a means of positive identification for the corpse in a safe place for the authority's use after the conclusion of the emergency. If the grave draws the attention of dogs or wild varmits, it is not deep enough. In this case, place heavy stones, bricks or concrete blocks over the grave to keep animals from disturbing the remains.

Exhumation after the emergency

Once the emergency is over, you are required to notify the authorities about any deceased people you buried. They will need to have the details about the person and their manner of death before a death certificate is issued and the body can be exhumed and reburied in the cemetery or cremated. In rare instances, the coroner may wish to perform a post-mortem examination on the deceased in which case they will be responsible for recovering the body from the burial site. In most cases, however, this task will fall to the local mortician who is likely to have a backlog of bodies to attend. For instance, the British Government reported that burials could be delayed by 16 weeks during a moderate pandemic.[95] If the pandemic is severe, the wait will be even longer. So it will be important to bury the dead well because they may need to reside there for quite a while before being moved to their final resting place.

CHAPTER 13

Essential Water and Food Supplies

The pandemic period is likely to last about 18 months, during which intermittent interruption in the commercial and public infrastructure may be common. [20] Complete recovery from widespread dysfunction in the economy may take longer than anticipated, perhaps extending well beyond the end of the official pandemic period. No matter where you ride out the pandemic, that place needs to be properly prepared and stocked with essential survival items. A stash of three months of essential supplies should last through the time when supplies will be most difficult to obtain. General Preparedness

Once the pandemic starts anywhere in the world, the U.S. Government says it will reach your town within a month, plus or minus a few weeks. Now, before the pandemic begins, you still have time to plan and purchase items your family will need. While influenza pandemic appears increasingly likely, the timing of it is uncertain. Since the world has been in *de facto* Pandemic Phase 4 since the summer of 2005, as discussed in a previous chapter, *now is the time to begin obtaining essential supplies.* This gathering includes, at a minimum, all the items on the Flu Survival Kit, your basic food rations, water storage/collection containers, and the items included in the Spartan Energy Plan

Since the world has been in *de facto* Pandemic Phase 4 since the summer of 2005, now is the time to begin obtaining all your essential supplies.

Water

Minimal water requirements

At a minimum, you will need two gallons of clean water each day for every member of your family. This quantity is just enough for the primitive cooking, drinking, cleaning, and sponge bathing of one person. You will need to supply enough storage container capacity to provide this minimal level of water for at least one month. This calculation assumes a reasonable prospect of being able to refill your containers from a reliable source several times each month. If this is unlikely, then you should plan to have two or three months of storage capacity available. A large margin of error is desired when it comes to something as crucial as clean water. Water

Living on two gallons of water per day is going to be difficult for most people. A fugal bath in a small tub uses between 10 and 20 gallons or water. Adding a bath once a week for everyone will increase your minimal water storage requirements by 2.5 times. For each person in the family, the water storage capacity would rise from 60 gallons to 150 gallons.

Simple water recycling

You can reduce your consumption of water by simple recycling. Two or more people can share bath water. Another idea is to reuse bath water for clothes washing, then again for dishwashing, and, finally, for watering the garden. If you wash the items in recycled water and rinse them in clean fresh water, you can maintain hygiene. What's more, if you had a large solar still, you could recycle your water after all these uses into clean drinking water again. This option is particularly appealing for those living in an arid region where the prospect of resupply is unreliable.

Water storage

Water storage choices are multiple. One of the easiest methods is in 30-45 gallon refuse containers widely available from hardware stores. You can also purchase new high-density, polyethylene tanks in various sizes up to 500 gallons or used multiple 55-gallon tanks suitable for water storage. Water

Make sure the container you purchase is new, or at least cleanable, and suitable for storage of potable (drinkable) water. Don't buy a used container that held toxic materials previously, as these toxins will leach out of the plastic into the water for months, even after a thorough cleaning. Drums suitable for drinking water storage are indicated as appropriate for "potable water" use. Used drums that contained food or beverage products are excellent choices as long as these "food grade" plastic drums are sufficiently cleaned and disinfected. Original Articles

Place the containers where you want to store them before filling. Once the containers are full of water they will be too heavy to move; as water weighs 8 lbs per gallon. Also, the weight of the water stored in containers could cause structural damage to the building so carefully consider their placement.

Water sources

If water utility service is disrupted, you will need to find a reliable, clean water supply to refill storage containers. Possible solutions are rainwater, surface water, and solar stills. Since this supply is so important, you should decide early how you are going to accomplish replenishing water, setting up your system before the pandemic begins. Once Phase 6 of the pandemic is realized, fill all your water storage containers with clean water from the tap. Books

Rainwater collection

If you live in a region of the world with regular rainfall, collecting water that falls on your roof may offer the best solution for you.

Water Collection and Storage

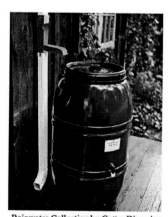

Rainwater Collection by Gutter Diversion

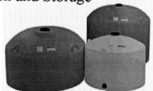

150, 300, and 500-Gallon Water Storage Tanks

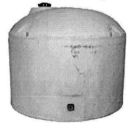

1500-Gallon Water Storage Tank

You can make your own rainwater collection set-up using a gutter elbow and flexible plastic pipe shaped to fit in the gutter. Use these supplies to make a gutter diversion kit that fits into the downspout from your roof. This set-up will allow you to divert water running down the spout into the plastic pipe, then into a large container. Window screen material can filter the rainwater before it enters the container.

There are several ready-made rainwater diverter kits that are nice with useful features. Several online retailers sell these units both with and without barrels.

If you plan to use rainwater as your primary water source, clean out and scrub your gutters now while you still have water service. Wash them down thoroughly with 1:10 bleach solution to get rid of the bacteria and protozoa. A high-pressure washer is very useful for this chore. <u>Original Articles</u>

Keep your roof and gutters clean of debris from this point on. If the barrel has a spout attachment, it will be useful to elevate it 3 feet off the ground. This way, when you attach a garden hose to the barrel, you will have sufficient water pressure to use the water a considerable, horizontal distance away. In case you never need to use your rain barrel water system as a potable water source; you can always use it to water your yard or garden, especially if your area is experiencing a water shortage.

Water from rivers, lakes, springs, and streams

In rural settings, even surface water that appears clean may be contaminated with bacteria and protozoa like Giardia, especially when located in areas of the woods inhabited by wildlife.

In agricultural areas, water runoff is often polluted with pesticides, herbicides, fertilizer, and animal wastes, including chicken manure in some areas that could contain bird flu virus. The water may look, smell, and taste fine but still be contaminated.

In urban settings, most creeks, rivers, and streams are contaminated with E. coli bacteria from leaking septic and sewage systems. These waters are often polluted with chemicals from yard runoff or industrial sources. The water may or may not look drinkable, and it will often having a slight odor and polluted taste. Surface water near industrial areas may contain a number of toxic chemicals. Chemical contamination causes the water to have an odor, be discolored, and/or have a bad taste. In general, don't trust surface water. If it looks, smells, and tastes good, collect it, but don't use it until you have purified it. If the water looks, smells, or tastes bad, avoid it completely.

Natural spring water can be fine as long as the water does not surface farther up the spring bed before dipping back underground. Scout above the source and make sure that this cause of contamination is unlikely. A covered cistern at the head of the spring is the best way to collect water. The cover keeps leaves and animals from gaining access to the water in the cistern.

Water purification methods

Unscented household bleach

Plain unscented household bleach is the most practical way to purify a large quantity of water. For adults, the Federal Emergency Management Agency (FEMA) recommends adding 1/8th tsp of household bleach to each gallon of drinking water to get rid of virus, bacteria, and protozoa.[96] This treatment is unsafe for infants until it has been run through a good filter. Allow the water to sit for 30 minutes after adding the bleach before consuming or using it.[97] <u>Original Articles</u>

Water Purification and Filtration

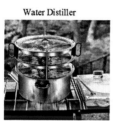

Water Distiller

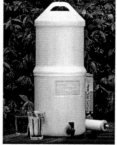

Solar Powered Floating Ion Purifier

Gravity Feed Activated Carbon Water Filter

Water filters for removal of particulates and chemicals

For cleaning, you can use water purified with bleach without further treatment. The portion you plan to use for drinking or cooking needs one additional step to bring it up to class "A" water standards. You should filter the purified water through a system that removes particulates and organic and inorganic chemicals. A good choice are the pitcher-filter systems sold by Brita® or GE®. These tabletop units use an ion exchange resin plus activated charcoal to remove all impurities from water. These filter methods are limited to filtering about ½ to 1 gallon at a time. If you choose this method, buy several extra filter cartridges, and you may want to have more than one pitcher device, too. These filters are available in the kitchen section of department and discount merchandise stores. <u>Water</u>

Boiling

If you have enough fuel, the FEMA recommends boiling water for purification.

Solar still

Consider constructing a solar still, which removes contaminants through distillation. This method is one of the only practical ways to desalinate seawater for drinking. To do so, you will need a flat reservoir to hold the unpurified water, a glass or clear plastic cover for the reservoir, and moderate handyman skills. These devices can produce quite a bit of clean, distilled water on a bright sunny day any season of the year.

Solar water disinfection

A clever and inexpensive way to purify water is by use of the solar water disinfection technique (SODIS).[98] This low-tech simple method can purify small quantities of water quickly and cheaply. In essence, to purify water with this method simply fill a 12, 16, or 32-ounce clear plastic bottle commonly used for soft drinks about half full with clear but unpurified water. Clear means free of particles or cloudiness but not purified. Place the bottle in full sun for at least 6 hours, preferably upon a corrugated metal sheet. The ultraviolet light from the sun and the heat generated in the bottle both work to purify the water within.

To clear up turbid water, filter it through a cotton cloth first then use sedimentation to clear up particulates floating in water. Sedimentation means filling a clear container with water and letting it sit for a day of two. Most of the particulates will settle down into the bottom of the container. Use a siphon to remove the clear upper layers of water from the container. Once the water is clear, it can be purified using the SODIS method.

What to do once water service is restored

Once water service is restored, officials recommend waiting at least 78 hours before drinking it. You can use the restored water service right away as long as you continue to use purification practices. Water that comes out of the tap immediately after the water service is restored is often contaminated with bacteria. Since it may be impossible to have an uninterrupted water service while the pandemic is underway, you should refill all of your storage containers as soon as regular water service comes back online. That way, if it goes off again, you will be prepared.

Basic food supplies

Stock up on foods that do not require refrigeration, are highly nutritious, can be prepared under campout conditions, taste good, and are reasonably priced. [99] A three-month supply of these basic foods will be sufficient to see your family through most worst-case scenarios. Food

Condiments, vitamins, and minerals

Your diet will be more interesting if you have a variety of key spices on hand for use during the emergency. The health of your family will be more secure by having a three-month supply of high quality multiple vitamins for each member. In addition to multiple vitamins, don't forget calcium for everyone and an iron supplement for female teens and women of childbearing age.

Recommended storage foods		
Common Name	Item	Food Group
Canned meat	Beef, chicken, ham, and fish	Protein and fats
Dried beans	Pinto, garbanzo, white, lima, black eyed, red, butter, lentils, and soybeans	Carbohydrates, fiber, healthy fats, and protein
Edible oils	Canola, sunflower, and olive	Healthy fats
Nuts	Peanuts, pistachios, cashews, almonds, walnuts, pecans, peanut butter, and sunflower seeds	Healthy fats, proteins, and carbohydrates
Dried fruit	Raisins, apricots, prunes, figs, bananas, apples, pineapple, and dates	Carbohydrates, minerals, vitamins, and fiber
Grains	Whole grain rice, wheat, and oats. Includes whole grain flour, grits, and crude bran	Carbohydrates, protein and fiber
Dairy	Dry fat-free milk	Carbohydrates, protein, and calcium
Eggs	Dried whole eggs	Protein and fat

Special food items

Don't forget to include special items such as candy, dark chocolate, powered lemonade concentrate, and brandy. These foods and libations will come in handy from time to time, especially when everyone needs a lift.

Vegetarians

Vegetarians will have little trouble following a beans and rice based diet. A good supply of spices, dehydrated onions, and vegetable bouillon cubes will ensure variety. Since fresh dairy and eggs are likely to be scarce, be sure to stock up on dry milk powder or canned milk, and powdered whole eggs if you are an ovo-lacto vegetarian. You can supplement your diet with these two sources of high quality protein. Preserved milk with a fairly long shelf life can be purchased in Mylar/cardboard containers. The milk tastes fine, but its price is high. Dry milk, while slightly less flavorful, is nonetheless as nourishing and much more affordable.

Home gardening

An important food source of which most people can partake is a *home garden*.[92] Urban residents will be surprised at how much food they can produce with only a little bit of space, even a balcony. For suburban and rural homeowners, cold frames, tunnels, and greenhouses can extend the growing season year around. Having a garden will provide you and your family with an excellent source of delicious, fresh, and healthy vegetables, a precious commodity if foods stores close. If your group has access to a favorable spot, consider sponsoring a common garden. Gardening

There will be plenty of time to get at least two, if not three, bounteous crops from your garden given the expected length of the pandemic. Some of the food you grow can be perseeved for use later in the year. A guide to a variety of low-tech food preservation methods can be found in the Resource section of the BFM.com website. There are also several books that deal with this topic in the Pandemic Preparedness Store. Food Preservation, Books

Gardening

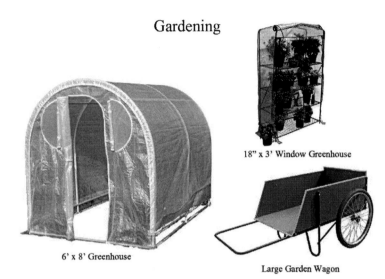

18" x 3' Window Greenhouse

6' x 8' Greenhouse

Large Garden Wagon

CHAPTER 14

Alternative Home Energy

Because there are so many options regarding alternative energy, you can spend many hours studying this issue and still be unsure which to choose. After careful thought, there were several that made a lot of sense to me. These are the ones presented here. They all share the characteristics of being practical, efficient, relatively simple to pull together, and reasonably priced although far from bargain basement. Complex high-cost solutions are not included here. I discarded these along with a plethora of charts, graphs, and formulas in favor of simpler options that will be good enough to see you and your family through the pandemic period. They will, however, fall short of your present access to power and heat. If the solutions here fail to meet your needs, consider consulting an alternative energy expert for further help.

Practical ways to meet your family's energy needs			
Energy need	**Recommended solutions**		
Home electricity	PV Panels with 12 V deep cycle battery array and backup Generator		
Space heating	Woodstove	Passive solar	LP gas heater
Cooking	Woodstove	Solar oven	LP gas stove/grill
Water heating	Woodstove	Active solar	Passive solar
Lighting	Battery operated fluorescent and LED lanterns		Flashlights
Entertainment & News	AM/FM/SW radio	LCD TV with DVD player	iPod, Game boy
Communications	Walkie-talkies	Ham radio	Police scanner
Other	Laptop computer		

Electrical energy

Living on a Spartan Energy Budget

In the event of a power grid failure, you will need an alternative way to generate electrical energy. Without a power grid, people will have to restrict themselves to a *spartan energy budget.* In this no-frills budget there isn't room for most modern appliances like ovens, stoves, hot water heaters, clothes washers or dryers, dishwashers, freezers, refrigerators, and central heating and cooling. These big energy users are unsupportable under conditions with limited electricity. Envision these circumstances as camping out in your own home. Considering the average worst-case scenario we may be asked to cope with rolling blackouts or even a complete failure of the power grid lasting a month or two. If these events come to pass, you will need to adapt to a severely limited energy supply. As President Bush said in February 2006, "America is addicted to oil." True enough, but even more broadly we could say, "America is addicted to energy." <u>Alternative Energy</u>

Fortunately there are alternative energy solutions for almost everything for which we use electrical appliances today. This includes cooking, heating, and washing. It is costly to produce energy alternatively. Therefore, to keep your upfront cost down, plan to limit your family and yourself to the bare necessities as you formulate a spartan energy budget. A simple solution designed to satisfy your basic needs will be better than a complex solution fulfilling your desires but at great expense.

Possible energy solutions

The best approach calls on a combination of methods. Where you live, the amount of money you can spend, and your basic energy needs also define the solutions from which you will choose. For instance, the approach advocated here for home heating begins with improving the energy conservation performance of your home, dressing properly for cooler conditions inside your home, making use of passive solar heating when available, and using a small woodstove or a back-up LP gas heater to keep a small room warm during winter. Photovoltaic (PV) panels, a bank of deep cycle batteries, an AC inverter, and small back-up gasoline generator can help meet electric needs. Hardware, Books

Home electricity generation

How much electric energy do you need each day to meet your most basic domestic needs? Don't be surprised if you have no idea. Most people don't and why should they? Today we live in a world where electrical energy is incredibly cheap and its supply virtually endless. These circumstances have promoted and supported a national lifestyle that wastes this precious resource and takes it for granted. But to return to the question at hand, how much electricity will you need to meet your basic requirements? The easy answer is a lot more than you will be able to produce through alternative means.

Our personal use of electrical energy is quite astounding when calculated. Take a look at your electric power bill. Most people will find it a challenge to produce only a quarter of the power they consume each month. The common answer then is to plan for a dramatic reduction in electric energy use.

You can easily calculate how much energy you need to support your basic electrical energy requirements. Start by making a list of every essential item that uses electricity that you will need during a prolonged power grid failure. Strike any big energy consumer now; it will save you time later and help you begin to come to terms with how really limited your energy supply will be. Next determine how much electricity each of these items consumes and how long you will be using them each day. This information is then converted into watts, a useful unit of energy. The watt is measure of power used by a device over a specific time, usually one hour of continuous use. It is also a way of expressing the amount of useable energy available from a power source. The formula for calculating watts is:

Watts = Volts x Amperes

Some low power devices like the iPod or Game Boy use the term milliampere (mA). There is 1000 mA in each Ampere. Most electrical devices contain a plate that lists the voltage and amperage or wattage. Wattage on a device indicates how much power is consumed by it when used continuously for one hour. So, a 100-watt light bulb will consume 100 watts of power each hour it is on.

To calculate how much energy you will need to operate a device, simply multiply the number of watts it requires by the average length of time you use it each day. For example, if you want to keep a 13-watt compact fluorescent bulb lamp on for three hours per night, the energy required would be:

Energy (Watt-hours) =13 Watts x 3 hours = 39 Watt-hours per day

After gathering the information on each of the items on your list, you are ready to cast your spartan energy budget. In the accompanying table, a truly bare bones energy budget is projected for a family of four. Notice that this budget provides enough energy for basic lighting, a radio, and some short-range walkie-talkies. Even this very minimal use of electrical energy will require the generation of almost 500 watts of electric energy each day.

"Bare Bones" Spartan Energy Budget spreadsheet for family of four						
Load	Rated Volts	Amps	Watts	Duration (Hours)	Number in Family	Daily Watt-Hours
Flashlight small 2AA	3	.25	.75	4	4	12
Flashlights Medium 2C	3	.5	1.5	3	1	4.5
Flashlights Large 4D	6	.75	4.5	3	1	13.5
Battery Lanterns 4D LED	6	1.25	7.5	8	2	120
Battery Lanterns 8D Fluorescent	12	1.1	13	8	2	208
Walkie-talkies	4.8	.7	3.36	8	4	108
AM/FM/SW Radio	6	.5	3	6	1	18
					Total =	480

Consulting with an alternative energy expert

The limiting factors for solar PV systems are access to sunlight, cost, availability of PV panels and their complexity, which rises with their electrical generating capacity. The ins and outs of even small PV systems are complex and one of the drawbacks of this approach. Another is the safety risk of working with a bank of 12 V deep cycle batteries, which is significant. This manual provides nothing more that the most basic outline of these systems. Bells and whistles too advanced for this manual do exist. For this reason, you should discuss your needs with an alternative energy consultant. If you plan to install a medium to large system, especially one that will have a tie-in with the electrical power grid as part of a permanent solution for your domestic energy needs, a private consultant is mandatory. For those interested in obtaining a small solar system as a temporary solution to the risk of a power grid failure during an emergency, the staff consultants at the Internet alternative energy vendors Real Goods and the Alternative Energy Store are excellent sources for expert free advice. These sources can help you better define your needs and help you get the most system for your money. They will specify exactly what equipment you need and help you set your system up properly and safely. They also can provide you with up-to-date pricing and product availability information.

Small photovoltaic solar systems

For many reasons, solar PV panels have some strong advantages. This alternative energy source has matured and is very reliable. The technology is stable, and the panels last at least 20 years. The cost per watt is about $5 for panels of 100 watts and larger but is much higher for smaller panels. If you have sufficient sunlight available, a small PV system is an excellent solution for most family's basic electrical needs in the case of a power grid blackout. Depending on where you live and weather conditions, having about 200 watts of PV generating capacity for every 500 watts of energy consumed each day provides most people with a significant margin of safety.

Basic Small Solar PV Based Power System

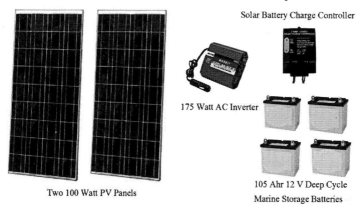

Solar Battery Charge Controller

175 Watt AC Inverter

Two 100 Watt PV Panels

105 Ahr 12 V Deep Cycle
Marine Storage Batteries

A basic system configuration involves attaching the PV panels to a charge controller that services a battery bank. The battery bank saves surplus power generated during the day for use at night or when cloudy conditions reduce your PV panel's power output. The power stored in the batteries is made available by connecting them to a device called an AC inverter. The inverter takes the 12-volt direct current (DC) electrical energy stored in the battery array and converts it into 120-volt alternating current (AC) electrical power used by standard plug-in appliances. Even small systems require placement of special DC fuses between all the devices to prevent injury or fire. It also will be important to monitor your batteries state of charge with a voltmeter. <u>Books</u>

Living with considerably less electricity will represent a major shift for people residing in developed and even some developing countries. We already have a shortage of PV panels in the United States due to increased domestic and international demand for these devices. Since the chances of your obtaining this equipment after the pandemic begins are poor, obtain your system now. It also is important to set up your system and learn how it works before you have to rely on it. Murphy's Law applies to all endeavors. If your system has problems, getting help later on may be difficult. By gaining experience with your system, you may decide that you need more power. Therefore, if there is time, you can obtain additional PV panels, storage batteries, or a back-up gasoline generator.

Storage batteries

Batteries are a key component of alternative energy systems because they help manage mismatched power generation and use. Batteries allow the energy from your system to be stored for later use. While PV panels are only able to produce energy during the day, energy use extends well into the night. Batteries are used to compensate for the mismatch between energy production and consumption. It is essential for an alternative energy system to employ a good quality battery array to manage this problem. Two or more batteries can be connected together to increase their storage capacity while keeping the voltage the same. Batteries are heavy, and for this reason, most people do better to buy three smaller 80lb batteries and connect them together rather than one big 240lb monster that are difficult to move around. Alternative energy systems use deep cycle batteries that are made to store and discharge energy differently from typical auto batteries.

Storage and Auto Battery Accessories

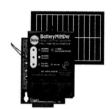

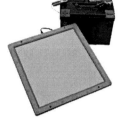

12 V Solar Battery Bank Charger

12 V Solar Auto Battery Trickle Chargers

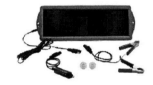

120 watt AC Auto or Deep Cycle Battery Charger

Deep cycle batteries

Typical auto batteries are a terrible choice for alternative energy systems. A good option for most beginners is a 12V deep cycle marine battery. A better battery is the 12V sealed gel cell deep cycle batteries. As premier beginner batteries, these are more expensive and not widely available at retail. Sam's Club and Costco offer the 12V deep cycle marine at a good value. Buy your batteries locally to avoid shipping charges. A reliable source and reasonable price for the sealed, and therefore maintenance free gel cell battery, is the on-line alternative energy dealer Real Goods.

Batteries are rated in different ways, including voltage, cold cranking amps, and amp-hours. They also are sold for use in autos, boats, golf carts, and for home energy systems. For all practical purposes, we only need to concern ourselves with deep cycle batteries that are rated at 12Vs. Avoid a battery with a cold cranking amps rating because most likely it is not a deep cycle battery and will not last through many deep discharges. The amp-hour rating is the number of amps the battery will release continuously for one hour at the given voltage. The watt-hr is the number of watts the battery can generate in one hour.

Volts x Amp-Hr = Watt-Hr

A rule of thumb for small systems is to have 200 amp-hours of 12V battery storage capacity for each 100 watts of PV panel generating capacity you deploy. This generalization may be inappropriate for you since the size of your battery array will vary according to the demands you will put on it.

Using batteries with alternative energy systems is a complex topic worth studying. Several good books on the care and feeding of batteries in alternative energy systems are highly recommended to anyone planning to install one of these systems. After completing your research, seek the advice of an energy consultant to discuss your options before buying. Books

Remember: these batteries are hazardous. Everyone has heard stories about how car batteries will occasionally explode. Inadvertently bridging the gap between the positive and negative poles of a battery array with a metal tool can create a fiery electrocuting arch of energy. The battery explosion will shower those nearby with sulfuric acid. So, treat your batteries with respect and always remember to act mindful around them.

Medium to large sized PV solar systems

These 500-watt-plus PV systems are more complex than the average handyman wants to tackle. The advantage of these larger systems is they can generate and store enough energy to provide you with a back-up energy source to operate most of your home's essential appliances. What's more, when these systems produce electric energy in excess of your needs, that power can be shunted onto the electric grid turning your power meter backwards. This type of hook-up is called a grid intertie and is one of the great advantages of a larger system. A problem with medium to large systems is their high initial cost as well as a low rate of return on investment. These systems are complex and require a consultant to specify the necessary equipment as well as an experienced installer. If you are interested in finding out more about these options, contact a private energy consultant or the staff consultants at Real Goods or the Alternative Energy Store.

Gasoline generators

Small gasoline-fueled, electrical generators are the best option for most homes needing a back-up power solution to a PV system.

Small Backup Gasoline Generators

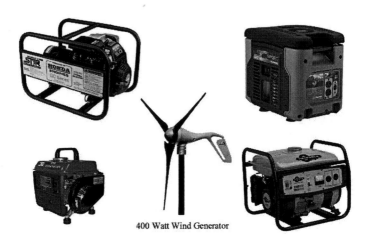

400 Watt Wind Generator

These devices have an output of between 1000 watts to 2500 watts, are fairly energy efficient, and have a reasonable up-front cost. The ideal situation is to use the generator to recharge your battery array when your requirements exceed the ability of PV panels. This approach will support regular use of power during an unusually long period of poor weather. It also is useful when you are at work on a special project that requires a heavier load on your batteries than normal. The generator will allow you to deploy a smaller PV panel and battery array adequate for your usual daily needs. For special needs, the portable generator can make up the difference. Hardware

Handy electrical devices

AM/FM/SW radio

A quality battery-operated radio capable of receiving AM,

FM, and short-wave stations will enable you to keep up with local and world events. There are crank radios and similar ones that have an attached solar panel are under-whelming when it comes to their ability to pick up distant stations. They are fine for local stations and are novel. The preferred choice is a good quality battery-operated short wave AM/FM radio because it has the power to bring in distant stations that might be out of reach of a lower quality crank or solar model. Electronics

Useful Electronic Gadgets

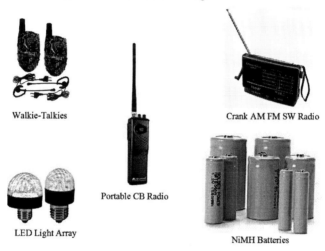

Walkie-Talkies

Crank AM FM SW Radio

Portable CB Radio

LED Light Array

NiMH Batteries

Having contact with the outside world will provide information about the status of the pandemic, developments around the world, entertainment, and survival tips. With the power grid down and most of our domestic radio and TV stations off the air, the short-wave bands will be a source of information from government emergency response organizations. Someone somewhere will be on air reporting the news and providing information of interest to flu survivors. Having the ability to receive news and even entertainment from Radio Australia will help people adjust psychologically to the stressed conditions. Accordingly, consider getting a good AM/FM short-wave radio. Electronics retailers and camping equipment stores are a good place to find these. Electronics

Flashlights

Each member of your family needs a small personal flashlight for use at night. They should be available at all times. These flashlights use two or three AA batteries. Good lamp choices include very bright halogens, and longer lasting, but not as bright, LEDs. The brightness of the halogen lamp can't be beat, but have a spare bulb or two because they will burn out. Most medium-sized flashlights use two or three C-type batteries and are very bright, especially with the halogen lamp. These are good work flashlights and useful for night repairs and security. The big 4D flashlights are too big and heavy for routine use, but they are capable of projecting a strong beam for quite a distance. Think of them as special purpose lights. They will be useful for situations where you need to put a lot of light on a big area or a spot that is not easily accessible. Lighting

Personal Lighting Options

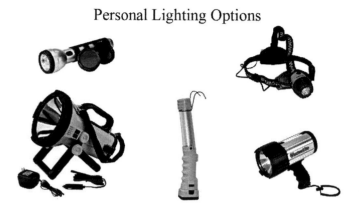

Shake-armature LED flashlight

A clever flashlight designer has developed a model with a sliding armature inside a wire coil connected to a small rechargeable battery in the handle. The flashlight charges itself when shaken back and forth. I was skeptical of these units at first but was pleasantly surprised when they turned out to be a dependable personal flashlight. They feature an LED bulb enhanced with a magnifying lens, which produces good light. Because they are such a new product, it is difficult to know how long they will last under regular use conditions. For this reason and because the superior brightness of the halogen lamp, the rechargeable NiMH battery-operated flashlights remain your most reliable option for personal lighting. This LED flashlight makes a good back-up and is an interesting way to teach children about power generation.

Pros and cons of LED, halogen, incandescent, and fluorescent bulbs

Both LED and fluorescent bulbs last much longer and use much less energy than traditional incandescent and the newer halogen lamps. The LEDs are five times and fluorescents are four times more energy efficient than the others. Flashlights with LED lamps use the least energy compared with halogen and incandescent bulbs. Halogen lamps produce the brightest and most intense light beam. Halogen bulbs are a little more costly than incandescent. LEDs will last for 10,000 hours, or virtually forever, while the others do burn out. Fluorescents last a long time too. However, all lamp types can and do burn out and some are simply defective. So, no mater which lamp type you select, have some back-up spares just in case.

Lanterns

When it comes to battery-operated lanterns, the best choices today are those that have LED or fluorescent lamps. The LEDs use less energy than fluorescent lanterns. The big fluorescent lanterns are great. Some, like the Coleman 13-watt 8D battery model, produce a light bright enough to light a small room well. This model is highly recommended based upon its low cost, ease of use, safety, and abundant light. Flashlights and camping lanterns that use LED are recommended for personal use while big fluorescent lanterns are best for general and task lighting. The LED lanterns are smaller and easier to carry around especially for a child. They can take the place of a small flashlight when walking through a dark house or on a path. The LED lantern is bright enough for reading, but most people will need to become accustomed to the lower light level. <u>Lighting</u>

Great Lanterns

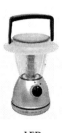
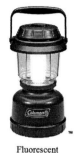
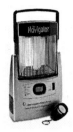

LED   Fluorescent   Fluorescent

Oil and kerosene lanterns

In the past, kerosene lanterns, oil-burning lamps, and candles provided indoor and outdoor lighting. These remain great standby alternatives today and are very reliable. Since fuel of all types may be scarce during the pandemic, be sure that you stockpile an adequate quantity of this fuel sources ahead of time.

NiMH batteries (AAA, AA, C, D, and 9V)

The common batteries used in radios, flashlights, and lanterns appear similar, but in actuality, they have many important differences. Most people are familiar with the disposable alkaline battery that works well until it runs out of power. The latest version of the rechargeable battery is a Nickel Metal Hydride cell (NiMH), a real improvement over past rechargeables. The NiMH rechargeable batteries are produced in the five common shapes and sizes (AAA, AA, C, D, and 9V) but not all store as much power as their alkaline cousins. NiMH batteries are nontoxic and can be recharged more than 500 times. The initial cost of NiMH batteries is substantially more than alkaline batteries, but the long-term cost is much less given the number of times they can be recharged. Electronics

NiMH has one important disadvantage; they loose about 10% of their charge each month whether used or not. Another issue is a limited availability of the "C" and "D" sizes, especially ones with a power rating similar to the same-sized alkaline batteries. In fact, several leading makers of the "C" and "D" NiMHs simply have taken an "AA" NiMH battery and repackaged it in a larger case. These then are sold as size "C" and "D" but only have the mAh of the "AA". You can get "C" and "D" NiMH with the just about the same mAh capacity found in the same-sized alkaline batteries with some searching. The best sources for the high-capacity NiMH are specialty retailers on the Internet. The price of these "C" and "D" NiMH batteries is higher than the low-capacity models, but the improved performance of these batteries is more than worth the extra cost.
Electronics

Small solar battery chargers (AAA, AA, C, D, and 9V cells)

A variety of small PV panel battery recharging options are available to charge NiMH batteries of all sizes. These units and chargers are specialty items and slightly more costly than others, and they are not widely available in stores. Internet-based retailers have been the best source for these devices. An important factor is the output of the embedded solar cells. With some low-powered solar battery chargers, charging 4 AA batteries could take all day. The last thing you want is to save $14 on a less expensive charger and then be unable to use a battery-powered device you need.

Portable AC power systems

The best use for these portable AC systems is to store power that you need to use at some distance from your principal battery array. These devices are essentially a battery and AC inverter combination. With it, you can take the power to the people. The portable battery can be recharged directly with a PV panel or by simply connecting it to your main battery array. This system is too small to meet the needs of most families alone. It simply does not carry enough juice.

AC Inverters and Portable Power Packs

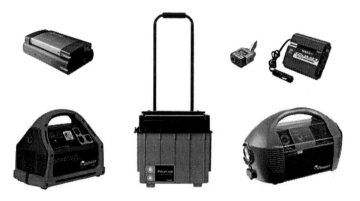

DC power packs

The problem with DC-powered devices is their reliance on a cigarette-lighter plug similar to the one found in most cars. You are unable to plug your DC light or fan into an AC outlet. So, you have to figure out a way to get power from your main battery array to another location in the house or yard where you need the energy. To overcome the distance challenge, you need a portable power pack with a DC outlet. These self-contained units are pre-packaged, small sealed, deep cycle, lead acid batteries that are connected to a couple of DC outlets and a small voltmeter. The combination is bundled into a container with a handle. Some of these units can be heavy to carry around so consider using a luggage cart. The portable battery pack can be recharged using the main storage battery array and taken to wherever you need the power. You also can run your AC appliances off it by plugging in an AC inverter. Electronics

AC Inverters

The AC inverter changes direct current (DC) made by alternative energy systems and stored in batteries into alternating current (AC) used by household appliances. The units are rated for how many watts of energy they can handle at one time. So, with a 500-watt inverter attached to battery array, you could connect and operate several small appliances as long as the total power consumed by them does not exceed 500 watts. Most households on a spartan energy budget will have their needs met with an inverter no larger than 500 watts. You will experience no problem hooking up a larger inverter or a combination of several smaller ones. Remember to keep your battery power storage capacity in mind to avoid damaging them by discharging them too far. Only plug in energy-efficient appliances to the inverter. For instance, a table lamp using a 13-watt florescent bulb will qualify as well as a charger used for a laptop computer or rechargeable flashlight. It is also important to learn how to monitor your batteries state of charge using a voltmeter. AC Inverters are available at auto supply stores, hardware stores, and online from Internet alternative energy sites. Electronics

CHAPTER 15

Home Heating, Cooking, and Hot Water

If the electric power grid fails, operation of furnaces that use fuel oil will be difficult, as will those that use natural gas or LP gas. The reason for this difficulty is that these appliances rely on electrical thermostats for control and electric fans to circulate air through the home. <u>Space Heating</u>

Home camping

Camping at home is a little like car camping, only much more luxurious. You get to sleep in a real bed, you don't have far to travel, and you have excellent shelter from wind, rain, and snow. What could be better? All kidding aside--approaching the problems presented by the pandemic with a sense of humor helps. There will be many similarities to "roughing it" except you will have most, but not all, the usual comforts.

Heating needs

Your heating needs are determined by where you live and how well insulated your home is. While you know the average temperature in your area, you may not know the insulation status of your home. Even if you think your home is well insulated, consider getting a home energy audit. Many utility companies offer these audits free of charge. Since most people will be riding out the pandemic at home, taking steps now to maximize your home's energy efficiency will pay big dividends later, particularly if you end up "camping out" in your home without power or water service.

The two most logical sources of alternative heating during a pandemic are either a small woodstove or one of several passive solar options in combination with a fossil fuel backup heat source. This portion of the manual focuses first on ways to reduce your home heating needs by improving its energy efficiency and by suggesting ways you and your family can be comfortable in a cool, or even cold, house.

Improve your home's energy efficiency

One of the best ways to stay warm in winter and cool in the summer during the pandemic is by having a well insulated home. Doing so will reduce your demand for conventional energy today and require a smaller amount of alternative energy to heat or cool the house during the pandemic. This is a smart move, with or without a pandemic, and something that you and your family can appreciate immediately in terms of enhanced comfort. It saves energy, adds value to your home, and has a good return on investment. Tax incentives may be available for theses energy saving enhancements from the U.S. and some state governments. The four areas where most homes can be improved include

- Attic insulation
- Insulated double paned windows with special coatings
- Insulated entry doors

- Carefully sealing areas around doors and windows where air can get in or out of the house.

Attic insulation

Blow-in insulation is an inexpensive and quick way to bring your home's attic up to modern standards. It can be placed in the walls as well as the attic. This is the single best way to improve your home's energy efficiency and will begin paying dividends immediately. Adding an adequate passive ventilation system for the attic to prevent heat build-up is also advisable with ridgeline vents being the most effective method. <u>Home Preparedness</u>

Insulated double paned replacement windows

Replacement windows offer many advantages over those originally installed in older homes. The new double paned insulated windows are designed to prevent the loss of heat in the winter or the gain of heat in the summer. The glass is coated with special materials that block heat gain while still permitting passage of visible light. The space between the two panes is filled with an inert gas that helps prevent heat and noise transfer through the window. Depending on the age and design of your present windows, the difference in performance experienced with these new windows can be dramatic. They are easier to clean and operate compared with older-style windows too. All in all they make a good investment as well as an excellent way to improve the quality of life for those living in the home.

Insulated entry doors

Makers of all types of doors have remarkably improved their construction and performance. The new high-tech doors are stronger than traditional ones yet weigh less. They are made of composite materials and sometimes metal and are insulated to prevent passage of energy or sound through its structure. There are many styles to choose from included those with double paned lights in them with the same advantages as the new windows. Replacing conventional doors with these new models will significantly decrease energy loss through this area of the home.

Sealing gaps and cracks around windows and doors

All gaps or cracks between the house and windows and doors or any other place in the outer wall of the home leads to an increase in energy requirements. Carefully inspect every door and window for these and eliminate them by use of insulation, caulk, or spray foam. Even small gaps between the door and the sill can result in significant loss of energy. If you are having your windows or doors upgraded, be sure and request that the contractor super-insulate the space between the window and the house to prevent energy loss from this area. Also, apply weather stripping or similar material around the door to reduce air infiltration around them.

Sensible clothing

Dressing for success here has a whole new meaning. While living in a cooler house than normal is not difficult, it does require forethought and planning. In 1978, President Jimmy Carter called for Americans to lower their home thermostats and wear sweaters indoors. While sweaters are still a fine way to stay warm, other practical and comfortable ways can accommodate a lower thermostat today. Layering of clothing is an effective and versatile method of living comfortably in a cooler house. Pandemic waves certainly can occur during the warmer time of the year but may be less common, as influenza prefers cold weather. <u>Clothing</u>

Clothes that can be washed easily by hand and that dry quickly on a clothesline will definitely make sense during the pandemic if we lose electrical power. Artificial fibers meet this need better than natural ones. Clothing made of polyester, nylon, and related materials wash well by hand in cold water and dry quickly.

Under-layers

Underwear technology has evolved since your grandfather's day. Long underwear today provides a wide range of performance capabilities, with undergarments appropriate for extremely cold to mildly cool environments. The thickness, materials, design, and manufacturing techniques of these garments affect their properties and provide the wearer with the exact combination of warmth, wicking (moisture evaporation), and material.

Clothing Suitable for Home Camping

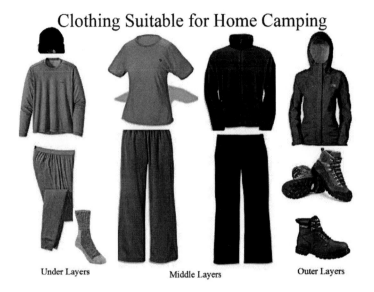

Under Layers   Middle Layers   Outer Layers

Middle-layers

Long and short sleeve T-shirts are commonly worn over long underwear. Shirts and blue jeans or other pants can be worn over long johns as a layering strategy. For more relaxed and comfortable attire, consider purchasing several lightweight fleece jackets and pants for use inside. Worn over the long undergarments, these fleece layers will provide warmth and comfort even in a cold house. They also can be worn outside as either an outer or middle layer. Fleece watch caps that cover the ears are a wonderful way to stay warm in a cold house, and these caps are great for sleeping, too.

Gloves and mittens

Hands can really get cold in a cool house. Working inside

with gloves is difficult, but several innovations offer solutions, gloves without fingertips, for one. These gloves have the last inch of the fingers removed so the wearer can manipulate materials normally. Another option is very thin, skintight gloves. These fine gloves make it easy to pick things up and manipulate them. A good strategy is to combine one of these approaches with a pair of fleece mittens that you tie to your belt with a string. When you don't need to manipulate objects, wear your mittens over the gloves. When you need fine motor skills, remove the mittens--an excellent compromise.

Warm socks keep your feet happy

The feet are the first part of the body to have reduced circulation when you get cold. The blood flow to the feet and ankles is relatively poor compared with the head, hands, arms, thighs, calf, and torso. So, feet need special attention in the cold. A good pair of thick socks is a good start. A number of affordable artificial fiber materials, which are almost as good as wool but dry faster, last longer, and cost less, are now on the market. A good choice for use inside a cold house and when sleeping is a pair of thick hiking socks that come up the calf, at least partway. The thicker the better when it comes to warm socks for inside use. Getting a pair of warm slippers to wear over the socks inside the house is a good idea, too. On a cold night, sleeping in a pair of thick socks can't be beat.

Outer-layers and boots

When working outside in the cold and wet, a waterproof but breathable hooded anorak is the best choice. Breathable means that water vapor released by the skin when working or exercising outside can pass out through the material while not allowing water or cold air to pass in. The anorak is worn over your fleece, and similarly constructed waterproof over-pants are also available. A pair of thick hiking socks inside a well-insulated and waterproof boot is a necessity if you are going to work outside in the snow, ice, or cold rain. Other outerwear options for working in dryer conditions include denim jeans and jackets. Don't forget to have a good selection of work gloves available to both protect your hands and keep the warm outside.

Sleeping bags

Sleeping bags have become very high tech over the last decade. The bags are rated by temperature so you can select one that is appropriate for the lowest temperature you are likely to encounter during the pandemic. Using a sleeping bag inside an unheated home could be an attractive option for many people especially children. Very good inexpensive options are available. The high cost bags are for campers who need lightweight bags they plan to carry in to a campsite. Great bags that weigh more are sold for a fraction of the cost of the high-performance lightweight bags. So the home camper can save some money but still stay warm. Inside Camping

Practical home heating solutions

The warm room concept

While it won't be possible to keep the whole house warm during the pandemic winters with no electricity, it is a very smart idea to keep at least one room nice and cozy. A good use of energy, this room will make a big difference in the quality of life and morale for everyone in your family. The strategy is to keep one room warm except when everyone is sleeping. This is where the family will spend most of its time when not sleeping, cooking, or working outside. For instance, if you use a wood-stove for heat, you should locate the stove in this room. Choose which room will become the future warm room now and begin thinking how you will adapt it for this purpose. If there is time, you can add extra insulation above the ceiling and below the floor. This is also the room where you want to provide adequate lighting. Light and warmth are very important ingredients to the physical and psychological health of everyone.

Woodstoves

Wood has been a reliable heating solution for humankind for thousands of years. While many think of the woodstove as a quaint device of historical interest only, as a technology, it represents the pinnacle in development of the art and science of wood burning that began when Prometheus first brought the gift of fire to our remote ancestors. The modern woodstove is one of the most efficient and effective ways to use wood for both heating and cooking. The traditional fireplace, while attractive, is a very inefficient method of heating, cooking, and warming water. In some cases, the draft created by the chimney takes more heat out of the house than the radiant energy from the fire adds to it. For this reason, fireplaces are not recommended as a routine heat source. <u>Space Heating</u>

Modern woodstoves come in many sizes and have a number of useful features including the ability to control the burning of wood by limiting the amount of air into the combustion chamber. This limit allows for varying the heat output of the stove to more closely match your needs. Woodstoves are affordable and can be inexpensively installed in an existing fireplace, or the flue can exit the home through a wall or ceiling vent.

The woodstove is good for cooking, space heating, and water heating--a versatility not to be found in any other single solution. The downside of a woodstove is its reliance on wood. It has to be stoked and lighted each day, and the ashes must be removed and discarded. Cutting wood for the stove is hard work and requires skill and some good tools. Having the right tools and stocking up ahead of time with an adequate store of seasoned hardwood is a good strategy for keeping your family well supplied for the winter. If you install a woodstove in your home and have access to a woodlot, this option may be the right one for you. <u>Space Heating</u>

Woodstoves

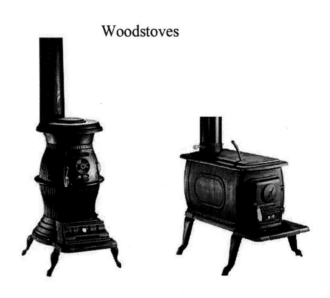

The solarium

Depending upon the orientation of your home to the sun, you may be able to add a solarium. While not a complete answer in itself, a solarium is a solution that has merit for some. While you may be unable to heat your entire house by simply adding a solarium addition, this passive solar option can make a big difference in your comfort when your conventional heating source is not functioning. The heat captured in the solarium is circulated through the adjacent portions of the house by convection, which depends only upon the difference in temperature between the air in the house and the solarium. Some clever solarium designs allow you to capture the daytime heat in a thermal mass for release at night. A solarium is an attractive long-term and cost effective solution to home heating. There are a number of companies that will design and build a solarium for you. These additions can be costly though, putting them out of reach of many people. A temporary solarium may be a viable alternative suitable for use only during the pandemic period for those with handyman skills. This solarium can be constructed using 2"x4" lumber and 4-mil polyethylene plastic sheeting. On the BFM website I have placed a plan for building one of these temporary structures in the Resources section under <u>Home Preparedness</u>. <u>Books</u>

Backup LP gas heaters

Small LP gas heaters have a low initial cost and do not require venting when used inside. They are safe and produce enough heat to warm a small- to medium-sized room comfortably. However, they use LP gas, which may become scarce and expensive during the pandemic. For this reason, these devices are best used as a backup heating method. As with any interior combustion heater, be aware that they can deplete the oxygen in a small room, potentially leading to death by asphyxiation. They come in various BTU outputs and use the widely available 20lb LP gas tank. Because these heaters use fossil fuel, if you plan to rely on this method, it would be wise to establish a stockpile of fuel before the pandemic begins. Using this heater in a backup role would be a nice fit for families that choose to use an LP gas grill as their cooking option. Both use the same fuel type so one fuel stockpile serves both purposes. Space Heating

Portable Backup Fossil Fuel Heaters

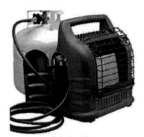
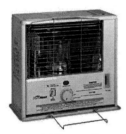

LP Gas Heater   K1 Kerosene Heater

Kerosene heaters

Another low-cost backup heating option are kerosene heaters. These make sense only if you have access to an adequate stockpile of the clean-burning K1 kerosene used by these heaters. The units used in the home range in output from 10,000 BTUs to 23,000 BTUs per hour. Oxygen depletion is an issue with these heaters, too. Another problem is incomplete fuel combustion that results in carbon monoxide release, which can also cause asphyxiation. The best use of this fossil-fuel-dependent heater is as a back-up heat source. Space Heating

Cooking

LP gas

All but the lowest end products of LP gas grills now come with a side stovetop gas burner and have dual controls for the main grill. The side burner permits you to heat food in a pot using a small flame as on a stovetop. The dual controlled grill allows you to broil using just half the grill. You can also bake in the grill by turning on only one of the burners and closing the top. You can smoke meat in the grill, a process that is energy efficient. If these options meet your cooking choice needs, consider purchasing one. Consider stockpiling at least two 20lb LP gas containers per person for cooking during the pandemic. Cooking

An LP gas operated camp or backpacking stove is also an appropriate cooking choice. LP gas burners without an attached grill are available, too. These burners are big and generate a lot of BTUs. They use significantly more gas than the efficient side burners attached to the LP gas grills.

If you plan to use LP gas for cooking and heating, consider buying or renting a larger tank in the 250- to 500-gallon range. You can refill the smaller 20 lb tanks from the larger ones using a special device.

Solar ovens

The sun's energy can be harnessed directly to cook your family's food. Solar ovens work very well on sunny days and poorly on cloudy ones so you will need to use them along with another cooking method. A good strategy is to combine a solar oven with an LP gas grill. There are several solar ovens models available, including plans for homemade ovens. <u>Cooking</u>, <u>Books</u>

Pandemic Cooking

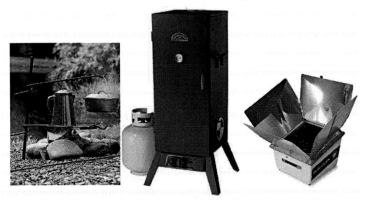

Open Fire Camp Stove   LP Gas Fired Meat Smoker   Sun Oven Solar cooker

Limited electric cooking

Those who have installed a medium-sized or larger PV solar system will have sufficient energy to operate a limited number of low-wattage electrical cooking appliances. Items that might fall into this category include a coffee maker or a crock-pot. For example, one family-sized crock-pot was found to have an energy consumption rating of 180 watts on low and 250 watts on high. This expenditure is reasonable as long as you have a renewable method of replacing this power. An advantage of the crock pot is its small draw of energy from your alternative system. These simple appliances don't stress the battery array, compared to an electric oven, microwave, or hot plate. These latter high-energy, high-demand, devices put considerable strain on a battery-based system because of the high current needed over a short time period to operate them.

"Fireless" cooking

Once a cooking pot filled with food has been heated to an appropriate cooking temperature, cooking will continue at just slightly below this temperature for quite some time if you remove it from the heat and place it in a highly insulated container. This is "fireless cooking", a technique taught me by alternative energy consultant William Stewart.[100] The fireless cooking container can be simply constructed out of anything from a cardboard box, laundry basket, or Styrofoam cooler. Place crumpled up newspapers in the bottom of the container and lay a terrycloth towels across these. Place the heated pot on this and then put more newspaper insulation around the sides and top of the pot. Cover this with more terrycloth and close the box. This is a great way to cook dried beans quickly using a pressure cooker. Place the beans, water, and a little oil in the pressure cooker and heat until steam begins to jiggle the pot's release value. Now the pot is ready to be placed in the fireless cooker. You can cook meat and bean soups in a pressure cooker this way too and very quickly.

Woodstove Cookware

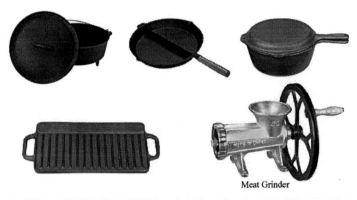

Meat Grinder

Hot water solutions

Solar hot water systems make dollars and sense now

Most homeowners use natural gas or electricity to heat water. Of all the alternative energy choices one has today, solar domestic hot water heating is the one with a competitive rate of return on investment. There are a host of off-the-shelf solar hot water solutions with proven track records, experienced installers, and even big tax credits for those who adopt this alternative whole-house solution now. You should consider doing this, pandemic or no pandemic. However, if you depend on city or county water, pandemic conditions may lead to a loss of water service, which will prevent you from getting hot water from your solar system.

Hot water during the pandemic

The conventional methods for heating domestic hot water may be non-functional at times during an 18-month long pandemic, presenting a challenge for most people. No matter what methods you select, you are going to need a dozen or so plastic five-gallon pails with handles to move water around. Baths will be a family affair with a tub of hot water being too precious to pour out and refill for the next person.

Since clean water may be at a premium, the preferred method of bathing will be in a metal or plastic tub just big enough for sitting. This tub will use less water than a traditional bathtub and will also make it easier to siphon the used water out of the tub and back into 5-gallon pails to reuse to wash clothes and dishes and, ultimately, to water the garden.

Passive solar water heating

Passive solar systems use no pumps or powered controls to circulate the water or control the process. The principal mover in a passive system is the conversion of the sun's radiant energy into heat.

Camping-style solar hot water container

These camp shower devices are simply a black heat-absorbing plastic bag that you fill with clean water and hang in the sunlight during the day. Capacities range from 3 to 8 gallons, just enough hot water to take a nice "Navy" shower. The sun's energy striking the black plastic bag is converted into heat that is absorbed by the water within the bag. Unless you live in the tropics, or it is a warm spring or summer day in the temperate zones, using this device as designed is a waste because too much heat is lost to the surrounding environment. Placing the bag within a large cardboard box insulated with newspapers, open to the sun, and glazed with polyethylene plastic will significantly increase the efficiency of this device. <u>Water Heating</u>

Tropical cistern solar water heater

If you live in the tropics, you can heat water by placing it in a black, closed container in the sun. These simple collectors are used throughout the third world where the temperature never or almost never goes below freezing. Large, black plastic cisterns are usually located on rooftops. Even without glazing, they produce large quantities of hot water. The batch collector is similar in concept to the simple solar cistern except it is located in an insulated and glazed box.

Batch solar collectors

A batch collector is a simple solar water heater that can be constructed from materials purchased at the hardware store or scrounged from the neighborhood. These devices trap the sun's energy in an insulated glazed box and convert the high-energy ultraviolet light into infrared heat when it strikes a black painted water tank within.

The batch collector is simply an insulated box with a window on one side and a water tank inside. Batch collectors, which come in a thousand variations of many varied materials, share a common, basic structure. These units can produce 20 to 40 gallons of hot water on a daily basis and function independently of electrical power or running water. On the BFM website, you will find instructions for building a 40-gallon batch collector from new or recycled materials in the Resource section under Home Preparedness.

Thermo-siphon solar hot water system

A thermo-siphon hot water system is a simple approach to water heating without pumps, motors, or controls. As long as the storage tank is located above the collector plate, circulation through the thermo-siphon plumbing loop is realized by natural convection of hot water. When a collector plate absorbs sunlight, the UV light is converted into infrared heat that is then transferred to water in the collector. The heated water expands and becomes lighter than the heavier and denser cold water. While convection moves the hot water up through the system and into the storage tank, gravity and suction pull the heavier water down into the bottom of the collector to replace the hot water that has risen. These systems can produce a lot of hot water each day, but they are more complicated to build. Additionally, this type of system faces a significant freeze risk that must be taken into consideration. Books

Heating water on a woodstove

Heating water in large kettles or pans on top of a woodstove is another viable option for obtaining a small, but adequate, supply of the precious commodity. The woodstove is a great way to heat water for baths and cleaning. It is the only "triple play" alternative solution, in which you get space heating, water heating, and cooking all in one.

Cooling the home

Swamp coolers

Cooling your house without electricity can be a challenge. If you live in an arid region, then using a swamp cooler is an excellent choice. This device is a humidifier that cools the air by converting liquid water into water vapor. It takes energy to change the state of a substance from a liquid to a gas, and this energy is subtracted from the temperature of the air. Warm air entering a swamp cooler is cooled down as it exits on the other side. Although these devices are electrical, they are really just a glorified fan and therefore don't use too much power. You would need to have at least a medium-sized PV panel system to use this device.

Dehumidifiers

In areas where the relative humidity is already high in the summer, a swamp cooler would just make things worse. When the temperature is high in these areas, the air is already close to being saturated with water. Therefore, people have difficulty in cooling themselves naturally through perspiration from the skin surface, resulting in feeling sticky and hot. Dehumidifying the air is one of the principal benefits of air conditioning in the summer. Air conditioners both remove the water from the air and cool the air. A dehumidifier removes water from the air but produces heat in the process. Overall, the benefit of less humidity exceeds the disadvantage of more warmth, as most people find stickiness more troublesome than the temperature. A dehumidifier uses less energy than an air conditioner. For example, an Energy Star compliant dehumidifier rated at 65 pints of water removal over 24 hours uses 115 volts at 8.3 amps, which equals 955 watts per hour of operation. While the dehumidifier will not be running 24/7, it still consumes a lot of energy and is beyond the capability of anyone on a spartan energy budget. However, the high-end medium-sized systems or the large alternative energy systems can handle its load. General References, Hardware

CHAPTER 16

Personal Hygiene and Laundry

Personal hygiene

It would be prudent to have on hand a three-month supply of basic personal toiletries, including everything from toothbrushes to tampons. Economy size containers of baby wipes will help reduce the need for water for hand washing and freshening up. Whatever you do, *don't* forget toilet paper. Your hygiene preparedness should include several galvanized steel or plastic tubs of varying sizes--small for dishes, medium for clothes, large for bathing.

Dry toilet system

This alternative, camp-style toilet, which will be convenient if you lose water pressure, is simple to make. To construct two complete toilet systems adequate for the needs of a family of four you will need: (a) two toilet seats with lids, (b) four empty five-gallon plastic paint buckets with tops, (c) one 40 lb bag of Quick Lime, (d) two 2.2 cubic foot bales of peat moss, e) one roll of duct tape, and (f) two garden trowels. This quantity of lime and peat moss will last a few months if used wisely.

Attach the toilet seat to the top of the paint container using duct tape to secure it temporarily. You will need to remove the seat when transporting and emptying the full container. Mix some of the peat moss and lime together (four parts moss to one part lime) in one of the five-gallon containers and place it next to the dry toilet. Place two scoops of the peat/lime mix in the bottom of the container before use. After each use of the toilet, use the scoop to sprinkle some of the mixture on the excrement, just enough to cover it. This mixture will reduce but not eliminate the odor. Toilet paper is biodegradable and fine for use in the container. However, the container cannot accommodate paper towels or feminine hygiene products.

A good way to dispose of human waste is to bury it in a latrine trench. Dig a simple latrine that is 18" deep, 2' wide and 6' long. When the container becomes 2/3 full, remove the seat, put on the lid, and take the pail into the yard, pour it into the latrine and mix it with some compost. Then cover the mixture with a little of the dirt you excavated from the trench. Fill this latrine systematically beginning at one end. Finally, cover the latrine with chicken wire to keep animals from disturbing it. The night soil will completely decompose in a few months, becoming excellent fertilizer in the process. Clean out the pail, replace the seat, add two scoops of the lime/peat mix and the dry toilet system is ready for use.

Laundry

The process of washing and drying clothes will change dramatically if the electric grid fails. Washing clothes by hand in plastic or metal tubs and drying them on a clothesline will be the best option for most people. Liquid laundry soap for use in cold water will be an essential item. Ribbed washboards, used extensively to scrub stains out of clothes in the past, may make a comeback. Interestingly, this old-timey device works much better than modern washing machines for this purpose. <u>Cleaning</u>

Hand-operated clothes washers

For a few people, the Wonder Clean® a simple hand-crank laundry device, makes washing clothes by hand more efficient, requiring less work to get the job done. This small appliance is only able to handle a few lbs of clothes at a time. For this reason, it would fail to meet the needs of families well.

The James Washer® is the real deal. Representing the height of luxury for the modern women in 19th= and early 20th= century America, this family-sized, hand-agitated device is well made. It has a washboard accessory as well as a hand-operated roller/wringer that removes most of the water so clothes dry much faster on the line. It has lots of capacity, even more than most modern machines, so it should work fine for large families. After the pandemic, it will make a wonderful conversation piece!

Cleaning

Laundry

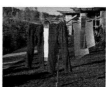
Umbrella Clothes Dryer

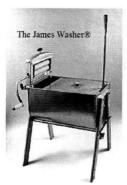
The James Washer®

Clothes Drying Rack

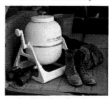
The Wonder Clean®

Table-Top Washing Machine

Clotheslines and drying racks

The clothesline is a truly superior way of drying wet garments. On a sunny day, clothes will dry quickly on the line. Sun-dried clothes smell great and get the purifying effect of UV light. An alternative to the clothesline is a clothes rack, especially in winter when you may be drying clothes inside to take advantage of the heat and to increase the relative humidity in the house. Both ways of drying clothes save energy and are well worth the few minutes it takes to hang clothes on the line or the rack. Cleaning

Home-made solar drying room

A solar drying room is another laundry option. The drying room also may serve as a home heating solarium if connected to the house through a door or window. This handyman project is constructed using 2"x4" lumber, 4-mil clear plastic, a staple gun, 16 penny nails, and a hammer. The dimensions of the rectangular drying room can vary to suit your needs, but for a single family, consider a 6' wide x 6' tall x 20' long room. Build the wooden structure first and apply the clear plastic with a staple gun to the outside of the 2x4s. If needed, apply a second sheet of plastic to the inside of the 2x4s to substantially increase the drying room's heat retention. A room this size will accommodate three clotheslines. Frame a doorway into the room somewhere near the middle of long axis of the structure. Fashion a door out of two overlapping flaps of polyethylene plastic. At the top of either end of the room, frame in a small window and fashion a flap of plastic to cover it. When the room is loaded with wet clothes, partially open the window and door flaps to allow dry air to enter and humid air to leave the room.

CHAPTER 17

General Family Preparation
Wills, insurance, and important documents

Make sure your will is in order and up-to-date.

Do you have enough life insurance? If not, now is the time to get more. Is the company you have insurance with the highest quality? I recommend you purchase insurance only from the bluest of blue chip companies because insurance industry studies predict that some companies may not remain solvent after the pandemic if their reserves are inadequate to cover the losses possible from a severe pandemic. <u>Pandemic Economics</u>

Another consideration is long-term disability insurance. Many people were disabled for years or permanently by flu or its complications during the 1918 pandemic. If you have this, see if you can have the payout indexed to inflation to protect the value of your benefit.

Do you have enough property insurance and is it a replacement policy of a fixed amount? A replacement policy is recommended because inflation could get out of hand during and after a pandemic. Make a complete written inventory of all your valuable personal possessions including furniture and appliances. Take current pictures of these items and the outside and inside of your home and any other insured property you own. Place a copy of today's newspaper in the picture scene somewhere so you can reliably date the state of your assets at least at that time. Place the inventory and pictures with your important papers. Having this documentation of your property will make it easier to establish your claim should your property be damaged or destroyed during the pandemic.

Consider pre-paying your property and life insurance policies or setting up a sufficiently pre-funded automatic payment method to cover your insurance premiums so that these payments can be made even if you or your family is not in a position to do so. This could happen because of illness or inability to make payments because of financial system dysfunction. This prevents the insurer from cancelling your policy for non-payment.

Where are your assets? Make a list of all your savings, checking, and brokerage accounts for your family or executor should this be needed. Where are the deeds to the property you own?

It is important to have positive ID for each member of your family. Do you have everyone's social security card? What about passports? Where are the children's birth certificates? It would be wise to obtain up-to-date and verified school transcripts for all the children and college students as well.

Gather all this information and the critically important legal documents. Make several copies of each and place the originals in a bank safety deposit box. Keep one copy with you and place the others with key family members or friends to preserve for your family.

Autos

If you are thinking about the purchase of another automobile, consider one that is fuel efficient, perhaps one of the hybrid cars now available. Since gasoline may become difficult to obtain, buy several five-gallon gas cans to stockpile gas. If you plan to use a small gasoline-powered generator as a backup for your solar PV and battery electric energy system, you will need a larger gasoline stockpile. In this case, consider purchasing a 55-gallon plastic or steel drum and a rotary hand pump to use for gasoline storage and transfer. Since having so much gasoline stored in an aboveground tank at your residence is potentially hazardous, don't fill the cans or drum until Pandemic Phase 5 is declared. <u>Fuel Management</u>

Fuel Storage and Management

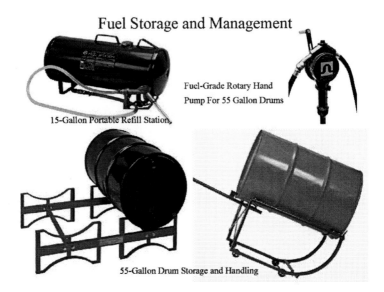

15-Gallon Portable Refill Station

Fuel-Grade Rotary Hand
Pump For 55 Gallon Drums

55-Gallon Drum Storage and Handling

In addition to fuel, install a new battery in your car; change the oil, the filters, and coolant. Obtain several bottles of gasoline stabilizer from the auto parts store. Pour this fuel additive into your tank when it is time to put your car up for the duration of the pandemic. You will also need to add fuel stabilizer to any gasoline or other liquid petroleum product you stockpile for use during the pandemic. Each product uses its own type of stabilizer. Buy a solar trickle charger for each of your vehicles to keep their batteries from running down. These plug into the car's 12V female outlet (cigarette lighter) and keep the battery fully charged even if you don't operate the vehicle. Once phase 5 of the pandemic is confirmed, fill your car's tank with gas and keep it full from then on. This will also be the signal to begin depositing gasoline in your stockpile. Don't forget to add the fuel stabilizer.

Battery Powered Electric Bicycles

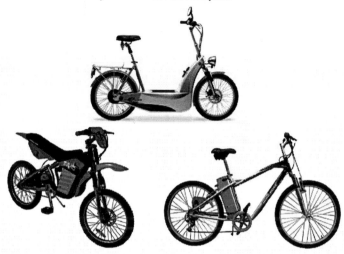

During the pandemic, you will probably not be doing very much driving. If the economy is shuttered by the pandemic, you will have fewer reasons to drive, so conserve your gas. Many people will not be working. Schools will be closed, and it is uncertain how authorities will interpret social distancing policies, as it applies to shopping in malls or Big Box stores. Gasoline will be hard to find and expensive. If your car is new or in good shape, consider purchasing a cover to place over it to protect its finish during the time you have it in storage.

Driving also may be unsafe during periods of civil disorder and reduced law enforcement. However, you should start your car and drive it around the neighborhood for a few minutes every few weeks to rotate the tires, circulate the oil and gas inside the engine, and give the battery a jostle. Driving outside the neighborhood could be dangerous, especially during an electric grid blackout or if police protection has deteriorated.

Useful items from the hardware store

Nylon rope in small and medium diameters will come in handy for a variety of needs, including making a clothesline and constructing a temporary shelter. Plastic cable ties (various sizes) and duct tape top the list of handy items for numerous uses. Consider loading up on these items in large quantities. Contractor's contact cement in large tubes and wood glue will prove useful for building and repairs. Hardware

Buy several plastic tarps (12' x 12' minimum) for making emergency roof repairs, constructing temporary shelter, and keeping dry. Having several rolls of 4-mil or 6-mil polyethylene plastic 10' x 100' will prove useful, too. A roll of 24" aluminum roofing sheathing and aluminum cutting shears will have a variety of uses for the creative handyman during the pandemic.

To construct temporary structures during the pandemic, stockpile a supply of pressure treated 2"x4"x10' studs. This building material will be very handy for constructing a variety of temporary items and structures like a solar batch water heater, a solarium, or solar drying room, for instance. In addition, you will need a 16 penny nails, a hammer, saw, and staple gun with several boxes of ½" staples. Several sheets of ½ inch plywood will increase your construction and repair options.

Tools

Obviously having a nice selection of hand tools will be important. If you are starting from scratch, purchase a ready-made kit that has everything you need in the way of screwdrivers and wrenches. Supplement this kit with a good hammer, handsaw, and crowbar. The most essential item to add is a 12- or 18-volt battery-operated 3/8" electric drill. This device is recharged using an AC inverter plugged into your battery array. With the power drill, you need a collection of bits--sold in large kits in different sizes and types for use on wood, metal, and concrete. The battery-operated hand tools are more expensive than ones using 120 AC house current, but if you have a PV panel power system with a battery array and a back-up gasoline generator, you should have no problem recharging this device. Usually, a good deal is to buy one of the kits the manufacturers sell that includes several commonly-used battery operated tools. Hardware

Battery Operated Tools, Tarps, and Bungee Cords

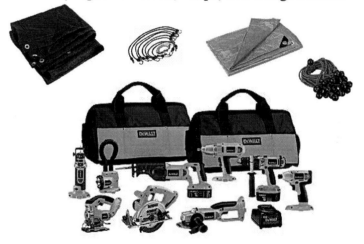

Firewood

As noted earlier, a woodstove is going to be a terrific solution for many because this single option efficiently provides for a family's home heating, water heating, and the cooking needs. Cut and split hardwood that has been dried for at least 12 months is considered properly *seasoned* for use in a woodstove. If you have the money, purchase a couple of cords of seasoned hardwood now. The wood must be carefully stacked on a sturdy frame to keep it off the ground. The stack should be covered with a well-secured waterproof tarp. Following these procedures will prevent your stored wood from rotting and help it maintain its fuel value. The wood will last several years or longer if maintained in this manner. Because this much wood is bulky, you will need sufficient space to store it properly.

An alternative is to cut and split your own wood. This approach requires access to a woodlot and the proper tools. It also is hard work, requires skill with tools, a woodsman's knowledge, and there is risk of injury. If you consider preparing your own wood, gather the correct tools for harvesting the trees, cutting the wood to length, and splitting it. Remember, wood needs to season for a year before use. Although unseasoned wood can still be used, the water content reduces its heat production, increases the smoke, and makes it harder to light in the woodstove.

Items needed include a good chain saw, axe, wood splitting wedge, and sledgehammer or maul. Several simple log-handling hand tools and a hand-operated hydraulic splitter are two options that make the task of moving and splitting timber less of a strain. Don't forget to obtain a good sturdy cart to move the cut logs from the woodlot to where you will be splitting them. You also will need extra gasoline and two-cycle oil for the chainsaw, lubricating oil for the chain, and several replacement chains. Pick up a chainsaw sharpening tool because using a dull saw blade is the fastest way to burn out your saw. <u>Hardware</u>

Harvesting Timber and Cutting Firewood

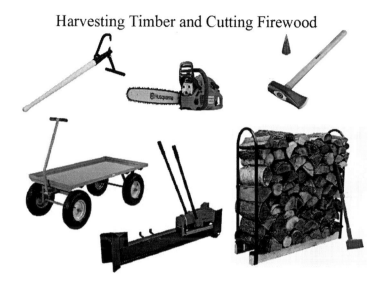

Communications

The commonly-available hand-held walkie-talkies that are rated for eight- to 10-mile range will be the best way to communicate with your family and neighbors if the phone system is not functioning. This rating is for line-of-sight distances only. If there are hills, houses, or trees between two of these devices, the effective range is approximately one mile or less. This range may be adequate to help keep up with your family members if they remain nearby. They will have a role in providing neighborhood security and emergency response. You will need to plug their battery charger into an AC inverter. Ideally, have at least one walkie-talkie for each family member and a couple of spares in reserve. Electronics

Powerful, long-range hand-held CB radios cost more but will allow you to stay in touch with people many miles away. Your family or PSG may wish to have at least one set of these to allow for long-range communications. For instance, a circumstance could arise requiring travel outside the neighborhood even when conditions are unsafe. The long-range radio can give you an idea of what to expect and what areas to avoid.

A CB radio base station will permit you to communicate with people near and far, but its operation will be dependent upon having a reliable source of power. These units usually require an operator's license, too. Some state and local authorities may use CB radios to communicate during the emergency. Having the capability to listen in on conversations both locally and from all over the world will provide you with information on how people near and far are coping with the emergency. Check with your local CB radio organization for more information.

Having a police scanner will be useful for keeping tabs on the types of crime and other problems the police are facing during the pandemic. It may give you forewarning of the activities of gangs operating nearby.

Useful household items

For repairs to clothing, shoes, and leather items, put together a good sewing kit with a variety of needles and thread. Pick up some extra blankets, such as soft acrylic blankets that are warm, easy to clean, and of great comfort value. Other useful household items include a supply of long-burning candles, at least 2-dozen disposable butane lighters, and several big boxes of waterproof matches and strike-anywhere matches.

Hunting and fishing

Nature provides an excellent source of high quality animal protein. It will be important to know how to properly butcher wild game and preserve the meat without relying on a freezer. I found several good sources of reliable information about this topic and have placed them on the BFM website Resource section in the <u>Food Preservation</u> area. Included are downloads covering butchering, drying, salting, smoking, and jerking wild game and fish. If you live in a rural area where hunting wild game is an option, be sure that you have an appropriate weapon and ammunition. If fishing is an option, pick up a variety of fishhooks, sinkers, and fishing line.

Entertainment

The spartan energy budget is unable to power TVs, DVD players, or X-Box video games. With a more robust alternative energy system, the extra power required by these devices could be accommodated. However, consider helping your family develop new forms of diversion. Frisbees, jump rope, toys, stuffed animals, and dolls promote play, as do puzzles and games. Parcheesi, chess, Scrabble, and checkers are reliable standbys. Card games like gin rummy, spades, canasta, bridge, go fish, cribbage, and poker are entertaining. Having a wide variety of games will be an important way to keep your children interested in these alternatives to TV. These forms or play and entertainment are superior to TV because they are active rather than passive, mentally challenging, and usually they are engaged in with other people rather than in isolation.

Reading will be an important activity during the pandemic. Have on hand a good supply of books that will last you for the duration. Consider branching out and trying something new like mysteries, or the classics or great books from the past-- Shakespeare, the Greek writers, and Roman historians. You can purchase many of these books in sets on eBay or at discounter retailers or used bookstores. These classic authors seem to improve with age – the book is the same, but the reader isn't.

Are you ready to home-school children K through 12?

Under pandemic circumstances, the government has announced plans to close schools. For this reason, if you have school-aged children you may want to consider home-schooling for the duration of the pandemic. Doing so will be the best way to ensure that your children will be able to receive an uninterrupted education of higher quality than possible from public or even private school. If you do elect to home-school during the pandemic and even afterwards, your children will have a much better chance of continuing their education uninterrupted during the emergency. If you are fortunate, a neighbor or friend may already be home schooling. This person can provide valuable advice to you. Some of the college students forced home by the pandemic might also be well suited and willing to help out with younger children's education during the pandemic. Home School

Home school materials are sold in complete packages that include textbooks, workbooks, homework assignments, tests, and a teacher's guide and course syllabus. There are several sources of new and used grade-appropriate home school materials from which to choose including eBay. You can purchase courses one semester at a time for one or more children. Look for opportunities to purchase home-schooling materials second-hand at a significant discount over new materials.

Mediums of exchange during the pandemic

Obviously, if the electricity grid is down, you will be unable to get cash from the ATM or bank. In the case of civil disorder or financial market closures, financial networks may be shut down. Merchants who can't authenticate accounts will not accept credit cards. If the banks close, no one will cash checks and everyone will want "cash money" or gold or silver coins. Unless prices are frozen by government action (which usually means, in practice, that goods become unavailable except on black markets, instead of just expensive), prices will skyrocket because of shortages.

Everyone's finances are tight. You probably think there is no way you could save a dime for the possibility of a pandemic. Fact is, most folks do have choices, and now is the time to begin establishing a cash hoard to see your family through this emergency. It is prudent to establish a cash savings cushion that is large enough to cover all your family's expenses for a 3-months. Put the money in a regular savings account at the bank. Vow not to touch the money not even for holiday spending. Make regular if not automatic payments into the savings account until you reach your goal. As soon as the Pandemic Alert Phase 6 is declared, withdraw all money in your account in denominations of $20 and $50 bills. This size bill is a good choice since black market sellers may not have the ability to make change for larger bills. You could stash your hoard temporarily in a safety deposit box but if your bank closes, your safety deposit box will be inaccessible. Consider preparing a good hiding place or two at home to keep your money and be sure to share this information with trusted family members or friends in case you are unable to access the money do to illness, separation, or death. Pandemic Economics

Small denomination gold and silver coins

If possible, use some of your savings to buy gold and/or silver coins and store them with your cash in a safe place. Small denomination coins will also be a useful item for trade. The U.S. Mint has issued a series of new 99% gold and silver bullion coins every year since 1986. They are called American Eagles and the gold version comes in sizes ranging from 1/10th ounce up to 1 ounce. The 1/10th ounce has a nominal value of $5 and is about the size and weight of a dime. Its market value is about $65 with the price of gold in the $630 area. Precious metal prices will probably rise if there is a breakdown in the financial system, but its value will be hard to establish because there will not be an efficient market to price it.

The small 1/10th oz coin should be very useful for trading during an emergency, and because it is a well-known US coin, it is self-authenticating as 1/10th oz 99% pure gold. The value of these coins will be higher than paper money, and there should be enough sellers willing to accept a recognized gold or silver coin in exchange for the scarce items. Platinum coins are also available and worth about 2 times as much as gold for the same weight. However, these coins are rare and less well recognized--a disadvantage.

The 1-oz 99% American Eagle silver coin has a nominal value of $1. Its market value is about $15 with silver bullion trading at $12 an ounce. This coin has utility at this value for trade. The weight of the coin is a disadvantage but not for making routine purchases.

When considering the virtues of these three precious metals, the 1/10th oz U.S. American Eagle gold coin is the preferred choice because it is well known, lightweight, small in size, and self-authenticating. Its $65 value provides sufficient purchasing flexibility when trading during pandemic times. The 1-oz American Eagle silver coin is also a viable option that should be included a cash stockpile since it will provide you with a smaller denomination currency when that might prove useful to have on hand while conducting commerce during the pandemic. A slightly less desirable silver coin option is the purchase of a bag of circulated U.S. silver dollars. They trade at about 23% discount to the price of silver bullion or $9,240 per bag with silver in the $12 range. These coins are sold at essentially their silver bullion value as they have no numismatic or collector premium added to the price. To make this more affordable, one thought is for several families to go in together and purchase a bag of these coins for use during the pandemic.

Barter

Simple bartering will likely be the preferred and most common method of conducting commerce during a civil emergency and afterwards for a period of time. Black market trading will become widespread once the government exacerbates supply shortages by implementing price controls that they will probably feel compelled to do. To the starving, a loaf of bread will be more valuable than paper money or gold because the bread will keep them alive today while currency and coins will not. Cash, gold, and silver will only be of value to those with a long-term prospective. These people will accept them in exchange for goods and services because they are well prepared until the eventual end of the pandemic when things will return to normal. The cash or gold price for high demand items like food, medications, flashlights, batteries, weapons, and ammunition will be extraordinarily high because of these critical life sustaining and protecting items will be very scarce. On the other hand, if you have a surplus of one or more of these scarce commodities, you will be well positioned to trade for other scarce items.

Crawl before you walk

OK, so you have a set of rechargeable NiMH batteries, a good LED flashlight, a solar battery charger, and an LED lantern. Great. Now what? Charge the batteries and start using them. How long does it take to charge the batteries with the solar charger? How long does the charge in your NiMH batteries last? How bright is the flashlight and lantern? Can you get around in the dark with the flashlight and read by the lantern? You will learn a lot from these tests. If you find the solutions you have selected are inadequate, you still have time to upgrade.

More power to you

What you will probably discover during this dry run is that the solar charger works but takes too long and delivers too little power for you to survive well. Most folks find they need more juice. They don't have enough light; need a radio for entertainment, and lots more of those expensive NiMH batteries with better and faster chargers. Very few Americans can get by on less than the 500 watt-hour/day spartan energy budget, and for this reason, you most likely will want a couple of 100-watt PV panels, a small charge controller, four 100 AHr deep cycle 12 V batteries, and a 300 watt AC Inverter. Hooking these sources of energy together requires simple handyman skills.

Battery safety is the biggest issue but don't let this alternative energy stuff intimidate you. While it is critical that you buy all these components now when they are still available, it also is important that you hook them all up and make sure that your small home power system works the way you thought it would before you need it. If you run into a snag, now is the time to discover it so you can consult a staff energy supplier where you purchased equipment. You also might decide to approach your needs differently or even look into one of the permanent alternative energy solutions like solar hot water heating or medium-sized PV panel, wind, or small hydroelectric options.

Drink a toast

What about water purification? Try mixing 1/8 tsp of bleach in a gallon of tap water, wait 30 minutes, then see what this tastes like. Then filter a quart of it through a counter-top Brita filter. How long does it take for the water to percolate through the Brita? How does it taste? Have you got your water collection containers situated and your method for obtaining replacement water nailed down?

Let them eat cake!

How about your basic food supply? Do you know what items you need and how much of each is required for three months?

Have you completed your buying list? Have you located your suppliers? Are you happy with your storage arrangements? Have you started rotating your food items? Have you experimented serving your family meals prepared from the stored foods? How about a cook-stove? How well does the solar oven work? How hot does the water get in the solar shower and can you really take a shower with just 4 gallons of water? It is a good idea to find out the answers to these questions before it is too late to make adjustments to your plan if needed.

CHAPTER 18

The Great Bird Flu Pandemic Begins

This chapter represents a look forward to what may happen during a Bird Flu Pandemic. While no one can foresee what will unfold, considering these possibilities now helps with the adjustment process later should they come to pass. For the purposes of this section, let us assume that H5N1 has achieved pandemic status, meaning that efficiently person-to-person spread of the virus has been detected. Once sustained human-to-human transmission of pandemic flu occurs anywhere in the world, the U.S. Government predicts that you will have no longer than one month to complete your final preparations before the first pandemic waves descends upon the United States.

Outbreak

The pandemic has begun in a remote region of the third world. The death toll is mounting, and the virus has reportedly affected large numbers of people living in one or two regional capitals. Television images show streams of refugees on foot fleeing the affected areas. The WHO is considering the declaration of Pandemic Phase 6. You are ready for the worst and hoping for the best. Your Pandemic Survival Plan was completed long ago and refined several times. Your Pandemic Survival Group has been working diligently to secure all essential supplies and is in the process of implementing the final preparations. You have prepared yourself physically, psychologically, and spiritually for the challenges of the pandemic. Now all you can do is wait.

<u>Worst Case Scenarios</u>

What to expect

The diversity of opinion on TV, radio, in newspapers, and on the Internet is astounding. Those paying attention will be whiplashed from the hopeful to the catastrophic. Instead of beginning their preparations, they find themselves glued to the TV, absorbed by a flood of information, the developing horror, and competing opinions. They are distracted and unsure what to do.

Confusion reigns supreme

Soon bird flu occupies everyone's attention. It is the big story in the news. By now, most informed people understand the potential for devastation inherent in a pandemic. Public health officials are mounting a major effort to halt the spread of the virus at its source. At first, they appear to be making progress but then new outbreaks are detected. The U.S. President implements travel restrictions into the country from affected regions of the world.

The media is filled with interviews with experts and public officials on the pandemic and its implications. The varied opinions and advice serve to confound more than inform. The wide and sometimes contradicting range of views expressed contributes to confusion of those uninformed about this issue, which includes the vast majority of people.

THE BIRD FLU MANUAL

The pandemic moves fast. It is spreading through the airways on the wings of jetliners. First come reports of flu in Hong Kong and southern Europe, then in Moscow, Paris, and London. Hospitals are mobbed by the sick and fearful in these cities. Schools and public gatherings are canceled and quarantines are imposed. Images of panic-buying overseas cause fear in other parts of the world where the virus has yet to appear like Japan and the United States.

Sadly, the vast majority of people where you live have made few, if any, preparations for the pandemic, and as they see the approaching nightmare, they scramble to catch up. Every grocery store is crowded with people quickly depleting the shelves. Desperate shoppers have thought little about what they need and are acting impulsively in their purchases. Fear is on the increase, and many people are confused and some are in panic mode. Irrational buying empties some grocery store supplies and fights break out in long checkout lines as consumers jockey for position. Emotions are running high, and the stress is clouding usually rational people's thinking.

The surge in buying affects retailers worldwide who are rapidly running out of many essential items. Drug store shelves are quickly emptied of cold and flu medications, aspirin, and cough syrup. Latex gloves and surgical facemasks are nowhere to be found. World stock markets are in a tailspin as money managers try to calculate the affect the pandemic will have on demand and supply of goods and services. The U.S. Federal Reserve lowers interest rates aggressively to calm markets.

Practical guidance

What should you do? Stay with the plan you have formulated and stand by those you plan to sustain during the pandemic. These two harbors are your true refuge in this pandemic storm. Avoid succumbing to panic and rampant emotions. Stay focused and complete your plan's loose ends. You know what's coming and are as ready as you can be for it. Sit tight and remain as calm as you can. Read a book.

Don't allow yourself to become glued to the TV and radio. Yes, you *need* to know where the pandemic is and when it will hit you, but too much time in front of the television or Internet screen means less time to finish final organization and preparation. It will only serve to confuse, unsettle, or upset you.

By virtue of having a plan to cope with this emergency and a reliable group of folks on whom you can depend to provide you and your family with help and support, you are well positioned to hold fast. While a severe influenza pandemic will be the most traumatic experience most people will experience during life, the simple plans you have made and implemented will be of immense value in helping your family and friends navigate many of the adverse conditions that are likely to occur. Despite great suffering, this emergency will end, and there is every likelihood that when it does, you and your family will have survived it. Bear this fact in mind at all times.

For those who take the pandemic seriously, the primary data point to watch for is *case fatality rate* for those sick with the pandemic strain. The US Government defines a severe pandemic as one with a 2% case fatality rate. The guideline I use to classify the severity of influenza pandemic is somewhat more conservative:

- Case fatality rate < 2% = mild influenza pandemic
- Case fatality rate >2% but < 5% = moderate influenza pandemic
- Case fatality rate > 5% = severe influenza pandemic

If the number of deaths exceeds roughly 5% of those who become ill with the flu, we are witnessing the beginning of an extremely severe influenza pandemic. A pandemic of this nature will have the direst effects on our society, resulting in terrible consequences. Having implemented a plan and knowing that you can rely on the members of your group to provide you and your family with support through the duration of the crisis, you have a major survival advantage. The vast majority of people will recognize neither that a dangerous pandemic has begun nor understand its ramifications. You will not waste precious time trying to understand what is happening or deciding who or what to believe. Instead, you will immediately act to execute the final portions of your Pandemic Survival Plan. Doing so will help keep you focused and sane.

Quarantine

If you plan to move to a rural area for the duration of the pandemic, do so before the flu reaches your region and certainly your city. Early during the pandemic spread within the United States, the DHHS Pandemic Influenza Plan calls for the imposition of involuntary quarantines as a means of containing the disease. If you hesitate, you might find the road out of town blocked by the state police or National Guard troops, or even the U.S. Army. So leave before you have to. Get situated and comfortable in your new surroundings.

If you have selected an urban retreat and get caught within quarantine, stay home and batten down the hatches. You should have anticipated this possibility in your plan. If you find yourself in this circumstance, keep your head down and stay put. Don't draw attention to yourself. Remain where you are within your prepared refuge. There will be no safer place for you or your family. You have what you need to survive the pandemic and hopefully are in a position to defend your family and the members of your group.

The quarantine will not last very long because it will not work. The disease will have already spread before the quarantine can be established. The police and solders enforcing the quarantine will soon come down with bird flu. Some will go AWOL because they have sick family members at home, or they have no stomach for using deadly force against fellow Americans. In short order, the quarantine will likely fall apart. Meanwhile, stay cool and keep your group together and unified.

The darkest night

At some point, probably at the height of the most severe pandemic wave, we will probably lose our electricity, water, and telephone service. Delivery of food, gasoline, and natural gas will cease, and the banks and financial markets will close. The reliability of police and fire protection will become uncertain. Under these circumstances, there could be riots and mayhem especially where people are concentrated and the shortages are greatest. The human mortality and trauma caused by a severe pandemic will be disastrous. However, it is impossible to predict the death and destruction stemming from a pandemic induced breakdown in civil disorder. Self Defense

Looters and roaming gangs of intruders could temporarily gain the upper hand, operating unchallenged in some areas. Interstate highways and many roads will be transformed into virtual parking lots clogged with abandoned cars and trucks. There will be many people on foot camping out here and there including in abandoned office buildings and department stores. It will be a little like the Great Depression with groups of hobos wandering around and Hovervilles sprouting up in the countryside filled with refugees from the unsafe cities. Bold highwaymen will rob the weary, and looters, home invaders, and deranged and starving people will all be wandering around. Many people could become seriously injured and killed as a result of rioting, police actions, and crime. Dead bodies will be commonplace.

A time of heroes, cowards, devils and angels

The pandemic period will be a time of despicable cowardice and amazing heroism. Just as we saw with Hurricane Katrina, selfishness will coexist side by side with compassion and sacrifice. No doubt we will find ourselves challenged by many and diverse trials. But they will eventually pass, and we will pull through. Society will reconstitute itself, and our institutions will return. Should the terrible events predicated here come to pass, they will only be temporary. Probably the time of greatest risk will coincide with the pandemic's most devastating wave or peak and could last for two or three months. During this period, civil unrest with various degrees of lawlessness may occur. If the Great Bird Flu Pandemic follows the script of the Spanish Flu of 1918, then the second wave will be the most severe, and during that wave, an infrastructure already weakened by the first wave could utterly collapse, leading to a temporary anarchy.

Recovery and renewal

For a while, we will be defenseless and humbled by one of humankind's oldest foes, influenza in its major pandemic manifestation. But we will bounce back. It is just a matter of time--so don't let these dark predictions cause you too much worry. They are written not to evoke despair but rather to give you a glimpse of one possible version of how the "worse case scenario" might play itself out. If these dire predictions come to pass, having read about them here will help prepare and empower you to more quickly shake them off and get on with the task of survival.

Recovery will begin a month or so after the pandemic's crescendo but is likely to be interrupted as one or more additional waves of disease that pass through the population. This will be more psychologically traumatic than medically serious. Some vaccine will become available by that time, and industrial, civil, and commercial recovery will be apparent even during the last wave. By then, most people who were susceptible to the bird flu will have already had it. Some will have died but the vast majority will survive and know that they are now immune. Those who have recovered from the flu will be eager to get on with life and work. They will not fear the disease because they know that they can't get this pandemic version of influenza twice. The return of law and civil order will be followed quickly by the return of the power grid and water service. Not long afterwards we can expect a resumption of media (TV, radio, and newspapers), telephone service, and the Internet. These events will herald the coming end of the pandemic and the beginning of the recovery.

First and foremost, you need to have faith that you and almost everyone you know will survive this. Yes, there will be many deaths and an overwhelming number of sick people. But the odds are good that most of us will make it. In the event of a severe pandemic unfolding as foreseen here, my estimate is two in five Americans will have been very sick with the flu and one in thirty of us will have died. The worse case is for one in two being very sick with the flu and one in twenty dying. Based upon this worst-case projection, each of us has a 95% chance of making it through successfully, especially if we start right now to make realistic preparations for coping with the coming influenza pandemic. These are odds you can live with.

The End…and The Beginning

RECOMMENDED SOURCES OF BIRD FLU INFORMATIONBOOKS

One of the most informative sources of information is the recent documentary about the 1918 Spanish Flu written by John Barry entitled, <u>The Great Influenza</u>. This excellent work chronicled the worldwide epidemic from start to finish and provided me with a new perspective on just how serious influenza can be when the conditions are right as they are today. What I found most interesting in Barry's book were the many first hand accounts of how the pandemic struck the US and the world and just how devastating the illness was. The total inability of our institutions to stand up to the stress placed upon them by the 1918 pandemic was particularly enlightening for me. Alfred W. Crosby has also written a highly regarded book on this topic, <u>America's Forgotten Pandemic: The Influenza of 1918</u>. Both books are widely available in bookstores and the Internet.

<u>How to Prepare for a Pandemic</u>, by William Stewart is an excellent book covering practical aspects of home preparation for the emergency. The chapters on food stockpiling and storage techniques and alternative energy are especially comprehensive and informative. The book is available on <u>www.amazon.com</u>.

Websites

One site that provides an encompassing picture of the Bird Flu is FluWikie (<u>http://www.fluwikie.com</u>). This site has a wide variety of useful resources and background information on the pandemic. It hosts an active and enlightening Discussion Forum that covers virtually every pandemic related topic almost in real-time. It is the all-round best website for pandemic flu information.

Medical scientists around the world are closely monitoring the situation in Southeast Asia and regularly make reports that are published in the medical, scientific and lay press. You can follow these reports best using the Internet. Use Google News service at www.google.com to search for articles relating to "bird flu". This is one of the best ways to keep up-to-date on what is happening with the virus. Another great site that collects every article published in English on pandemic influenza is the www.iflu.org website. I check this site every day to keep up on new information.

A site maintained and authored by Henry L. Niman, PhD, a virologist with a special interest in recombinant viruses like influenza, is www.recombinomics.com. He provides an excellent commentary on avian influenza events worldwide and usually has information on new developments explaining their significance before virtually any other site. His views are controversial, but I usually agree with them.

Another excellent source for commentary is Effect Measure, "a forum for progressive public health discussion and argument", http://effectmeasure.blogspot.com/. The sponsor, Revere, is a particularly well informed person with a strong understanding of public health issues and policy.

An extremely valuable resource for reliable information is the Center for Infectious Diseases Research and Policy at the

University of Minnesota, directed by Michael Osterholm, a major figure in pandemic preparation circles: http://www.cidrap.umn.edu/.

Nature, the international journal of science, has an avian influenza web page that has a collection of articles their staff has done on the developing pandemic over the last few years. This is a wonderful resource for anyone interested in learning more about past, as well as future, pandemic developments: www.nature.com/nature/focus/avianflu.

THE BIRD FLU MANUAL WEBSITE ANNOTATED DIRECTORY

Resources Section

Advanced Home Treatment

The texts included in this section are intended for medical professional's use as they are medically technical, and some of the techniques discussed could be harmful if employed improperly by an untrained person. Most every article written for doctors on flu treatment deals mainly with drugs and vaccines but not day-to-day management of the disease, which I assume is because our medical educators do not think it is required. There are no books on treatment of pandemic influenza for doctors. The other problem with the materials written for doctors is that they all presume that really sick patients will all be treated in a fully staffed, supplied, and equipped, hospital.

Food Preservation

This section is filled with information on how to preserve meat, fish, fruit, and vegetables without relying on refrigeration. There is extensive information on the preparation of venison from "field to table". Use of smoking, drying, salting, and jerking of meat is explained. Dehydration of fruit and making fruit and vegetable leathers are taught. Canning by boiled water and pressure-cooking is thoroughly covered by several fine articles.

General Preparedness

The materials selected for this resource are more general

in nature and, for the most part, do not even mention influenza. They come from the FEMA and other agencies. The materials are quite extensive and comprehensive. They provide a lot of valuable ideas for preparing to cope with a disaster but are focused mostly on coping with the short-term consequences of a regional emergency than a long-term generalized influenza pandemic.

General References

The materials placed here are of a miscellaneous nature. They are documents that I found of some value for preparing or coping with a potential pandemic but which did not fit easily within any of the other resources categories.

Home Influenza Treatment

I placed flu treatment guides and advice for consumers from other writers and agencies found on the Internet or elsewhere here. There are very few good guides. This is one of the reasons that I thought it was necessary to write about this topic myself. In my opinion, the material written for consumers is too simplistic because the writers tried to keep it simple figuring that medical doctors would treat really sick patients. So there is not as much depth to these guides as we will need, but there is still a lot of good information in some of them.

Home Preparedness

This section has a good number of sub-sections given the complexity of the topic. There is quite a lot of materials that I thought would be useful to people interested in home pandemic preparation and they have been saved for you here.

Influenza Drugs

This section includes a PDF of the Physician Desk Reference write-up on each of the drugs listed in the Flu Treatment Kit in the book. The pharmaceutical company calls this document the drug's "product circular" (PC). These U.S. FDA approved documents include key research finds on these drugs. This includes the drug's approved indications, dose, duration of therapy, safety warnings, and potential and actual side effects of the drug.

Influenza Virology

This resource section includes articles that provide background information about the influenza virus. A variety of important scientific publications from peer-reviewed journals are included here as a reference for your use.

Medical References

This section includes studies on the symptoms and treatment of patients with the H5N1 bird flu virus published recently in peer-review journals. There are also articles on diagnosis of the virus and some that cover the public health issues related to this disease and its management.

Official Pandemic Plans

In the past year, several agencies of the US and other governments and international health organizations have released proposals for controlling or coping with an influenza pandemic. Some of these are published here for your review. These plans serve as the government's road-map for their efforts to contain the spread of the disease across borders or, failing that, how they propose to manage the pandemic once it affects the population.

Pandemic Economics

Beginning in August of 2005, several thoughtful and fairly comprehensive papers have been written on how an influenza pandemic might affect the economy of individual nations and the world. It is interesting to note that the articles written lately have a somewhat more realistic view of the devastating affect a severe influenza could have on the Global economy compared with some of those written in 2005.

Pandemic Survivor Groups

It is my hope that families will come together with their friends and neighbors to form a mutually supportive network of people dedicated to the survival of every member of the group. I call these ad hoc collections of people Pandemic Survivor Groups because it is apparent to me that one of the best ways to make it through an event like a severe influenza pandemic is to become a part of one. You do not want to face a pandemic on your own, and it is very unlikely, in my view, that the conventional institutions that we rely on presently, or might hope to rely upon will be effective during an emergency on the scale of pandemic.

Pandemic Survival Plans

Surviving the unconventional circumstances we may find ourselves facing during a severe influenza pandemic will require careful consideration and planning. Our bounteous society provides us with a seemingly endless supply of essentials that make it possible to enjoy our current standard of living. A carefully prepared PSP is an important first step to comprehensively prepare alternative solutions to many critical items like electric power, clean water, food, and security that most take for granted today.

Worst Case Scenarios

Several writers have shared their nightmare scenarios for what might happen during an influenza pandemic. Others have written about their experience during emergencies that occurred in the remote and recent past. Both sources of information provide the reader preparing for surviving a pandemic with a dark view of humankind at our worst but one that we may well have to face if the worst comes to pass.

The Pandemic Preparedness Store

Alternative Energy

Big and small solar photovoltaic panels and their accessories are featured in this section of the store. Among the accessories include good charge controllers for batteries, the better-quality sealed gel-type 12-volt beginners batteries, and DC fuses.

Books

I have encountered a large number of books of potential value to those interested in preparing for an influenza pandemic. The topics range from wilderness medicine, food-stockpiling methods, passive solar heating, gardening, camping, and military tactics. As you can see, these topics cover a lot of territory and the ones mentioned are just the tip of the iceberg. These books have one thing in common. They all have the potential to be of value to you and your family trying to cope with conditions possible during a severe pandemic.

Cleaning

How are we going to wash dishes, bathe, and clean and dry our clothes with no running water, electricity, gas, or hot water? With difficulty is the correct answer but there are several low-tech affordable solutions and methods that will work well enough to get through this mess. The methods are shared with you in the Bird Flu Manual, and the tools you might consider buying are located in this section of the store.

Clothing

You probably don't need any more clothes. If we have a pandemic though, you might find that the clothes you have aren't as practical as you would wish. Are your clothes easy to wash by hand in cold water and will they dry quickly on a clothesline? Do they lend themselves readily for use in a layering strategy that makes it comfortable living in a cold house during the winter? There is a whole line of clothing designed for use by active folks, travelers, and campers that fulfill these requirements and I have places them in this section of the store.

Cooking

There are several sensible cooking solutions for use if our conventional source of electricity and natural gas is not available. These include solar ovens, LP gas grills, and camp stoves. Believe it or not, there are a lot of manufactures of hand-operated appliances that require no electricity. You might find some of these kitchen items very useful to have around even if the pandemic is not the bear we fear it might be.

Electronics

Here is where you will find a few good AM/FM/SW radios and the hard-to-find high-capacity rechargeable NiMH batteries in all sizes. A selection of AC inverters and mobile DC and AC power centers (batteries on wheels) are found here. I have also included the short range walkie-talkies and a few long-range handheld CB radios, battery chargers, GPS devices, and many other useful gadgets can be found in this part of the store.

Food

This is where you can hook-up with vendors who sell dry goods to consumers in bulk. This includes wheat, rye, rice, corn, and dried beans. These suppliers sell these items in quantity, some in bulk unpacked and others in smaller quantities already packed for stockpiling. They also sell the materials used for long-term food storage including 5-gallon HDPE buckets with tops and handles, Mylar bags, and oxygen-exclusion devices.

Fuel Management

Your family or PSG is going to need to stockpile some fossil fuel for use during the pandemic when access to gasoline, diesel, LP gas, and kerosene could become very limited. It is tricky and potentially dangerous to store large quantities of these items in residential areas although they are routinely stored safely on farms and commercial establishments. The safe handling of these materials requires you to have a few basic tools including an appropriate container, fuel pump, hose, and fuel stabilizer to prevent its deterioration during storage. These are all found in this part of the store.

Gardening

Having a vegetable garden during the pandemic makes sense whether it be in containers on your balcony or in your backyard. It is easy, relaxing, and satisfying to grow nutritious and great tasting fruits and vegetables. These items may make the difference between surviving well and just getting by during the pandemic. Whether you are a beginner or an experienced gardener, I think the items you find listed in this section of the store will be of interest to you.

Hardware

Having the right tools and materials available will be critically important to cope with a number of potentialy adverse conditions occurring during the emergency. These range from a simple tool kit to special items like those needed to cut down tress and turn the timber into firewood. The range of tools, materials, and supplies that could be of use coping with the fallout from an influenza pandemic can be found in this section of the store.

Home School

Even if the pandemic is only moderate in severity, the authorities are likely to close public and private schools. Since pandemics last 12- to 18-months and come in 2 or 3 waves during that time, schools will be closed, then opened, then closed etc. The quality of education therefore, is not likely to be good. A workable alternative is to prepare to home school your children beginning at the start of the pandemic and continuing through the duration. This is one way to prevent them from losing a year of two of critically important education to the pandemic. Resources for this purpose can be found in this part of the store.

Inside Camping

While writing the Bird Flu Manual, it occurred to me that one way to look at the conditions that may prevail at times during the pandemic are analogous to camping out within our own home. Approaching the problem in this way helped me find several practical and easy-to-implement solutions to several problems that we are likely to confront as we try and cope with life's needs during the pandemic period. Items that you might find useful in this regard are located in this part of the store.

Lighting

Flashlights are much better these days than in the past. They are brighter, lighter, and tougher. The best flashlights of all sizes that I could find along with a good selection or lanterns that feature halogen, LED or florescent lamps are found in this section of the store. I have also included some battery powered florescent and LED work-lights.

Self-Defense

This topic is one that is pretty scary to many folks who just don't want to think about the possibility of large-scale civil disorder breaking out during the pandemic. We all hope that this does not happen, but it is clear that a lot of folks are concerned about this possibility. While it is not possible to predict what might happen, where, or how long it will last, this is a risk that has some probability of occurring and one that can and should be considered in our pandemic plans. Items potentially useful for this purpose have been displayed in this part of the store.

Space Heating

Keeping warm during the pandemic winter could become a great challenge should we loose the power grid and natural gas service. There are several solutions to this problem that are practical but not always inexpensive. Combining a long-term solution like a passive solar solarium with a portable LP gas heater is the type of solution that is likely to be effective but not available to most folks. Several solutions identified for this purpose are found in this section of the store.

Water

Water management during the pandemic is an issue because of the vulnerability of our municipal and county water systems to a power grid failure. It is essential that you have on hand enough potable (drinkable) water for you and your family for at least 1 month. In this section of the store you will find unconventional ways to collect, store, purify, filter, and distribute water to meet your domestic needs during the pandemic.

Water Heating

Hot water will be essential for bathing and cleaning. Access to hot water will become a luxury during the pandemic should our power gird fail. There are ways to heat water that do not rely on the power gird, and these solutions are provided in this section of the store. In addition, the commercially available solar hot water systems that make sense now for homeowners in many parts of the world are also displayed here.

Original Articles

In this section of the website I have placed a collection of articles written on pandemic related topics. They include monographs I have written on topics from pandemic politics to food stockpiling. Several articles provide a more in-depth exploration of topics covered in the Bird Flu Manual. Others are unique. My intention is to use this venue to publish new information on the pandemic as the need arises. Here is a partial list of articles currently available.

A Failsafe Pandemic Response Plan for State and Local Governments

The pandemic plans currently in place at all levels of government may turn out to be inadequate to cope with a truly severe event. The 2 million US deaths projected by the US DHHS Pandemic Influenza Plan in their "severe pandemic scenario" is not the worst case by any means. In my view, a better description of these estimates is the worst case they can possibly hope to cope with. A local plan that limits its worst case to this projection will have the same chance of succeeding as a levee built for category 3 hurricanes has of withstanding a category 4 storm. A truly severe pandemic is likely to have wide-ranging effects on the medical, social, and economic life of our country whose force will overcome these plans just as Hurricane Katrina spilled over the levees in New Orleans in August 2005.

Constructing a Homemade Steam Tent

Inhaling warm steamy air helps a variety of respiratory disorders. These include croup, bronchitis, and pneumonia. It is also useful for treatment of patients with thick bronchial secretions that are having trouble coughing them up. Using a steam tent is an appropriate way to provide this treatment to patients who need it.

The tent itself is constructed out of clear 4-mil polyethylene plastic. There are two simple designs. The first is for a *square tent* that sits at the head of the patient's bed covering the upper part of the body. This design is constructed using twelve 1"x2"x3' pieces of pine wood, 4-mil polyethylene plastic, duct tape, nails, scissors, hammer, handsaw, and a staple gun. Alternatively, the structure can be made using 1 inch PCV pipe. The second is the *tepee tent* that is made from polyethylene, string, and duct tape. It is suspended with string from the ceiling above the patient's bed.

Illness and Death During the Pandemic

When presenting how many people may become ill or die during a pandemic, one runs the risk of looking heartless. Statistics do not capture the uniqueness of each person, or the value of their lives. Rather than being an exercise in insensitivity, by understanding how serious the pandemic may be is necessary for making appropriate plans. No one is "only" a number; but numbers matter. For instance, knowing how many patients will be seriously ill during a pandemic affects the number of staffed hospital beds that will be needed.

Infection Control and Water Purification Using Household Bleach

Bleach is a strong and effective disinfectant. Its active ingredient, sodium hypochlorite, kills viruses, bacteria, mold, fungi, and protozoa on contact by denaturing their vital proteins. Bleach is effective, inexpensive and widely available making it a good choice for use as a disinfectant and purifier. Unscented household bleach is recommended because it can be used for water purification, disinfection, and cleaning. In the US, household bleach usually contains 6% sodium hypochlorite.

Home Gardening During the Pandemic

An important food source that many can take advantage of during the pandemic period is a *home garden*. Gardening is a satisfying pursuit that anyone can learn to do. Urban residents will be surprised at how much they can produce with only a little bit of space, even in a container garden on a balcony. Having a small garden will provide your family with an important source of delicious and nutritious fresh vegetables. Whether you live in the city or the country you can grow quite a few healthy summer and winter vegetables that will be important sources of variety for the diet.

Influenza Virus Evolution and Adaptation

The influenza pandemics of 1957 and 1968 were mild compared to the devastating 1918 flu. Studies show that genetic reassortment between avian and human flu strains led to the creation of the viruses that caused both these minor pandemics. In contrast, the 1918 pandemic virus adapted to humans by way of mutation and recombination. This alternative method of adaptation to humankind may contribute to the lethality of the virus because our immune system is less ready to deal with it. Another unique feature of the 1918 Spanish flu was the presence of killer gene segments (lethal polymorphisms). These gene segments are associated with widespread organ failure and damage not seen during the seasonal flu or the minor pandemics. Disturbingly, it was discovered recently that not only was H5N1 bird flu following the same evolutionary path taken by the 1918 virus, it had also accumulated many of the same lethal polymorphisms found in Spanish Flu. These observations are among some of the reasons to think that if bird flu achieves pandemic status it will be a man-killer on par with the 1918 strain.

Economic and Financial Implications of an Influenza Pandemic

A truly severe pandemic similar to the 1918 Spanish Influenza occurring at any time, but especially under today's circumstances where the human population is both highly concentrated in urban areas and enriched with many elderly and infirm persons, is likely to result in a human catastrophe. A medical disaster, disrupting commerce and civil order thoroughout the world can only result in grave economic consequences. The advent of globalization and interdependence of the world's economies means that adverse effects occurring anywhere in the world have significant impacts everywhere. Economic contraction due to a loss of production and consumption during and after an event like this is a predictable consequence. Future productive capacity will be impaired due to the death or incapacitation of a portion of the work force at all skill and professional levels. These events are likely to cause a fall in the value of many asset classes leading to further reduction in personal consumption due to a negative wealth effect. Several years will probably be required for the overhang of these fundamental factors to be worked off by the economies and GDP growth and capital markets recover.

Patient Triage During Pandemic Influenza

One thing that is different about a major pandemic is just how hard it hits patients and how rapidly it kills. Patients affected by the flu can be broadly categorized into 3 prognostic types. In medicine the term *prognosis* means the likely outcome for the patient with the disease. Patients with a good prognosis are expected to recover, and those with a bad one probably will not. How can I give you a prognosis on a patient I have never seen before? This is a medical skill that comes with experience, evaluating thousands of patients over the course of many years of practice. It comes from understanding the natural history of the common chronic diseases, and how they interact with acute infectious diseases like flu.

Support for a Personal Tamiflu Stockpile

It is responsible and ethical for physicians to prescribe Tamiflu for their patients to stockpile and use later during a possible Bird Flu Pandemic. Presently the risk of an influenza pandemic is high. The severe shortage of Tamiflu, the lack of an effective H5NI pandemic influenza vaccine, and my lack of confidence in the ability of the government to respond to an emergency on the scale of an influenza pandemic are all critical factors in my choice to support the practice of prescribing Tamiflu to patients for private stockpiles. Nationally there is a woeful lack of preparation to respond to this serious public health issue. My position differs from most government and medical bodies who have expressed an opinion. In this brief paper, I provide the rationale for why I think it is both practical and ethical for doctors to prescribe, and patients to obtain, Tamiflu prior to the pandemic.

Food Stockpiling Tips

Stock your pandemic pantry with foods that do not require refrigeration, are highly nutritious, taste good, can be prepared under campout conditions, and that are reasonably priced. These characteristics are ideal for use during the adverse conditions possible during a severe pandemic. I suggest you obtain a 3-month supply of these basic foodstuffs for each member of your family

Why stockpile 3-months of food for each family member? This quantity of food should be enough to see you through times when food is scarce. Since the pandemic is expected to last about 18-months, having a 3 month stockpile implies that you will still need to have access to food sources during this time, a prospect that is very likely. What is also likely, though, is that food shortages will occur from time to time during the pandemic period. During these time points, it will be difficult to find certain types of food. Your stockpile is intended for use during these times of scarcity. When supplies become more plentiful, restore your depleted stockpile. This way, you will be able to keep your family fed during the pandemic and not spend countless hours waiting in line for a handful of rice and beans.

The 1975 Swine Flu Debacle

The consequences to bureaucrats who needlessly warn the public about flu pandemics that fail to occur are seared into the US CDC's institutional memory. In 1975 an American solder stationed in the US died of influenza and an evaluation proved the organism responsible was HINI Swine Flu, a strain that was similar to the one that caused of the infamous 1918 Spanish Influenza that killed 80 million people worldwide.

CDC experts predicted a severe pandemic was possible and put on a big push to vaccinate the nation. At that time there were over 20 licensed influenza vaccine manufacturers in the US, so it was relatively easy for them to significantly up production from their usual order of about 50 million doses to 150 million. President Ford put his prestige behind the vaccination campaign by inviting TV cameras into the oval office so the nation could watch him get his shot. Speeches and public service announces were made imploring one and all to get a flu shot.

The negative experience of U.S. Public Health professionals and vaccine manufacturers during this debacle has been one of the reasons for the slow U.S. response to the bird flu emergency.

ABOUT THE AUTHOR

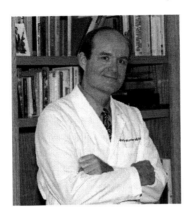

Grattan Woodson, MD FACP obtained his MD at the Medical College of Georgia in 1980 and completed his internal medicine training at Mary Imogene Bassett Hospital in Cooperstown, NY, an affiliate of Columbia University College of Physicians and Surgeons in New York, New York in 1983. He joined the full-time faculty of Emory University School of Medicine where he taught internal medicine and worked as a diagnostician at Emory Clinic.

In 1986 he left Emory to pursue a career in internal medicine and clinical research. His areas of expertise include osteoporosis, osteoarthritis, and Women's health. Since that time, Dr. Woodson has participated in over 50 clinical research trials and has been the principal or co-author of papers for peer-reviewed journals in the area of osteoporosis and metabolic bone disease, including the New England Journal of Medicine. He maintains his relationship with Emory University, where he serves as a Clinical Instructor of Medicine. Presently he is an attending physician in Internal Medicine at the Druid Oaks Health Center and the Medical Director of the Atlanta Research Center and the Osteoporosis Center of Atlanta.

Dr. Woodson first became concerned about avian influenza after learning about the first human cases in Hong Kong in 1997. His interest increased significantly when the disease re-emerged in Southeast Asia in 2003, a fact he discovered while researching the value of influenza vaccination in the fall of 2004. As the disease evolved, he became convinced that the likelihood of a worldwide influenza pandemic similar to the devastating 1918 Spanish Flu was increasing. To prepare his patients for a catastrophic event that many thought inconceivable at the time, Dr. Woodson authored his first book on the subject, *The Bird Flu Preparedness Planner*, published in November 2005 by HCI Books, Deerfield, Florida. The book was a success because it presented the risk we face from a bird flu pandemic in the clear and easy-to-understand style used by Dr. Woodson to explain medical issues to his patients. The success of this effort led to his writing the second book on this topic, *The Bird Flu Manual*, which presents a more comprehensive treatment of the topic.

REFERENCES

Endnotes

[1] "The pandemic flu virus in humans is most likely to be a mutation of avian flu virus H5NI" Lee Jong-wook, MD, the late Director-General of the WHO quoted in Internal Medicine Report, November 2005.

[2] Webster RG, Peiris M, Chen H, Guan Y., H5NI Outbreaks and Enzootic Influenza. Emerging Infectious Diseases • www.cdc.gov/eid • Vol. 12, No. 1, January 2006 (Influenza Virology)

[3] Walker K., WHO Possible bird flu pandemic not exaggerated. UPI 24Jan2006

[4] Hawkes N., Vaccine for bird flu may be useless say experts The Times 14Feb2006

[5] Peiris JSM, Yu WC, Leung CW, Cheung CY, Ng WF, Nicholls JM, et al., Re-emergence of fatal human influenza A subtype H5NI disease. Lancet. 2004;363:617–9.

[6] Avian Influenza: assessing the pandemic threat. January 2005 – WHO/CDS/2005.29 (Official Pandemic Plans)

[7] The Next Influenza Pandemic; Are We Ready? IOM Nov2004 (General References)

[8] Potter, CW., A history of influenza. J Applied Microbiology, 2001; 91: 572-579. (Influenza Virology)

[9] Plague of Athens 430 BC., Wikipedia 28Mar2006 (General References)

[10] Monto AS., The Threat of an Avian Influenza Pandemic 2005 N Engl J Med 352;4:323-325. (Medical References)

[11] The WHO Global Influenza Pandemic Plan July 2005 (Official Pandemic Plans)

[12] Olsen SJ, Ungchusak K, Sovann L, etal,. Family Clustering of Avian Influenza A (H5NI) Emerging Infectious Diseases • www.cdc.gov/eid • Vol. II, No. II, November 2005 (Influenza Virology)

[13] Ungchusak K, etal., Probable person-to-person transmission of avian influenza A (H5NI) N Engl J Med 2005; 352:333-40. (Medical References)

[14] Niman H,. Human Bird Flu Deaths Increase to I2I in Qinghai China http://www.recombinomics.com/ 25May2005

[15] Fact sheet: Information about Pandemic Influenza DHHS CDC 8Mar2005 (General References)

[16] The Writing Committee of the WHO Consultation of Human Influenza A/H5., Avian Influenza A (H5NI) Infection in Humans. N Engl J Med 2005;353:I374-85. (Medical References)

[17] Fox M,. Bird flu virus survives for days in bird droppings according to WHO. Reuters 2IJan2006

[18] Spread of H5NI by Contaminated Water. WHO 24Mar2006 (Influenza Virology)

[19] Chan MCW, Cheung CY, Chui WH etal., Proinflammatory cytokine responses induced by influenza A (H5NI) viruses in primary human alveolar and bronchial epithelial cells Respiratory Research 2005, 6:I35 doi:I0.II86/I465-992I-6-I35 (Influenza Virology)

[20] Osterholm M, Preparing for the next pandemic., N Engl J Med 2005;352:I839-I842

[21] UK Health Protection Agency Pandemic Plan for Influenza Feb 2005 (Official Pandemic Plans)

[22] The US Department of Health and Human Services Pan-

demic Influenza Plan. November 2, 2005 (Official Pandemic Plans)

[23] United Nations, World Urbanization Prospects, The 1999 Revision.

[24] Cowell A., Older Americans Sicker Than the English Study Says. New York Times 2May2006

[25] Roylance FD., Bird flu could migrate to US. Baltimore Sun 5Mar2006

[26] Bird flu could spread around the world veterinary chief. AFP 24Feb2006

[27] Woodson, G., Bird Flu Preparedness Planner, HCI Books, Deerfield, FL., 15Nov2005. (Books)

[28] York G., China hiding bird flu cases Globe and Mail 9Dec2005

[29] Niman H., False negatives for Bird Flu. www.Recombinomics.com Commentaries. 5Jan2006

[30] UN Officials Join Turks To Investigate Bird Flu Deaths. US Dept State 9Jan2006

[31] Outbreaks of Avian Influenza A H5NI in Asia. MMWR 13Feb2004 (Medical References)

[32] Marshal M., Genetic analysis reveals H5NI endemic in Southern China, NewScientist 6Feb2006

[33] Official from Ministry of Health Reveals 2005 Human Case Figures for Avian Influenza Outbreak in China. Boxun 15Nov2005

[34] Branswell H., WHO says countries sharing too little bird flu data to assess pandemic risk. Canadian Press. 12May2005

[35] For more on this follow the link to the BFM website and read the Original Article entitled Bird Flu Hanky Panky in Asia.

[36] Tjandraningsih C., Indonesia health chief says bird flu suspected in 3 deaths. Kyoto News 15Jul2005

[37] Thorson A, Petzold M, Thi N, etal., Is Exposure to Sick

or Dead Poultry Associated With Flu like Illness *Arch Intern Med* 2006;166:119-123.

[38] Niman H., OIE Declares H5N1 Endemic to Indonesia, <u>www.Recombinomics.com</u> Commentary 31May2005

[39] van Riel D, Munster VJ, de Wit E Etal., H5N1 Virus Attachment to Lower Respiratory Tract., SCIENCE VOL 312 21 APRIL 2006 <u>(Influenza Virology)</u>

[40] Wade N., Studies Suggest Avian Flu Pandemic Isn't Imminent. New York Times 24Mar2006

[41] Germans panic and dump their cats as Serbia joins the bird flu list. Disease Infection News, 5Mar2006

[42] Niman H., H5N1 in Dogs and Cats, <u>www.Recombinomics.com</u> Commentary 14Feb2006

[43] Bird flu spreads among Java's pigs, Nature Vol 435|26 May 2005 390 <u>(Influenza Virology)</u>

[44] Keawcharoen J, Oraveerakul K, Kuiken T., Avian Influenza H5N1 in Tigers and Leopards Emerging Infectious Diseases. www.cdc.gov/eid ,Vol. 10, No. 12, December 2004 <u>(Influenza Virology)</u>

[45] Director of the Center for Infectious Disease Research and Policy, the associate director of the National Center for Food Protection and Defense, and a professor of public health at the University of Minnesota, Minneapolis

[46] U.S. DHHS PIP: Table 1 entitled *Numbers of Episodes of Illness, healthcare Utilization, and Deaths Associated with Moderate and Severe Pandemic Influenza Scenario.* <u>(Official Pandemic Plans)</u>

[47] Chronic sickness makes Portuguese vulnerable to bird flu, viruses. AFP 9Apr2006

[48] US experts expect to be overwhelmed by bird flu. Reuters 2Feb2006

[49] McKibbin WJ, Sidorenko AA., Global macroeconomic consequences of pandemic influenza, Lowy Institute, February 2006, <u>www.lowyinstitute.org</u>. <u>(Pandemic Economics)</u>

[50] Woodson G, *The 1976 Swine Flu Debacle,* <u>Original Article</u> of the BFM website.

[51] Corwin JA., Bird Flu Scientists Face Tough Challenges In Developing Vaccine. RFE RL 20Jan2006

[52] Reaney P., Sanofi bird flu vaccine trial encouraging study. Reuters 11May2006

[53] Hamilton DP., Avian flu may tax vaccine makers. WSJ 02Mar2005

[54] Tamiflu Product Circular, Roche Pharmaceuticals <u>(Influenza Drugs)</u>

[55] Isolation of drug-resistant H5NI virus. Nature vol:437 20Oct2005 <u>(Medical References)</u>

[56] Hayden FG., Antiviral Resistance in Influenza Viruses —Implications for Management and Pandemic Response. N Engl J Med 2006 354;8 <u>(Medical References)</u>

[57] Moscona A., Oseltamivir Resistance — Disabling Our Influenza Defenses. N Engl J Med 2005 353;25 <u>(Medical References)</u>

[58] Chapter 50, Oseltamivir; Mechanism of action and resistance., in *Goodman and Gilman's The Pharmaceutical Basis of Therapeutics,* 10th Ed., 2001 McGraw Hill, New York

[59] Probenecid Product Circular <u>(Influenza Drugs)</u>

[60] Craft JC, Feldman WE, Nelson JD., Clinicopharmacological Evaluation Of Amoxicillin And Probenecid Against Bacterial Meningitis Antimicrobial Agents And Chemotherapy, 1979 16;3:346-352 <u>(Medical References)</u>

[61] Sowunmi A, Fehintola FA, Adedeji AA, etal., Open randomized study of pyrimethamine–sulphadoxine vs. pyrimethamine–sulphadoxine plus probenecid for the treatment of uncomplicated Plasmodium falciparum malaria in children. Tropical Medicine and International Health, 2004 9;5: 606–614 <u>(Medical References)</u>

[62] Hill G, Cihlar T, OO C, Etal., The Anti-Influenza Drug Oseltamivir Exhibits Low Potential To Induce Pharmacokinetic Drug Interactions Via Renal Secretion—Correlation Of In Vivo And In Vitro. Studies Drug Metabolism And Disposition 2002 30;1:13-19 (Medical References)

[63] Relenza Product Circular (Influenza Drugs)

[64] ACCP., Diagnosis and Management of Cough: Evidence-Based Clinical Practice Chest, Jan2006

[65] The patients will find it much easier to drink fluids from a baby bottle, squeeze bottle, or using a straw during their illness than from a glass.

[66] Petroleum jelly will be useful for chapped lips, noses, and bottoms. It will help ease the passage of an NG tube if needed.

[67] Use cocoa butter to make rectal or vaginal suppositories. It is also an outstanding lip balm and great treatment for chapped or irritated skin of the nose or perianal area.

[68] Thermometers break so have more than one on hand. These devices are all electronic now.

[69] Use a teakettle for making tea and as a device for making steam for treatment of sinus and bronchial disorders.

[70] Buy this in the liquor store. One common brand name is Golden Grain® but there are others.

[71] Tamiflu is expensive costing about $200 for 20 tablets. If you have insurance, you will still pay stiff co-pay. We have found that most insurance carriers will allow you for 10 tablets for one co-pay but will not let you have 20 tablets at once. If you wait two weeks and go back to the drug store and request the second 10, they will give them to you but you will probably have to pay second co-pay. This is really a pretty good deal when you consider the retail cost of the drug. All the other prescription drugs are generic and not expensive.

[72] Bacterial infection includes: Pneumonia, sinusitis, and otitis media (ear infection) all of which commonly complicate influenza and most of the causes of which respond well the azithromycin. Azithromycin is a well-tolerated antibiotic that remains active in the body for 4 of 5 days after the last does. It has very few side effects. A second treatment course may be required to clear the bacterial infection but I advise you to wait for at least 4 days after completing the first course of therapy to see the full effect of the drug before taking a second round of it. Azithromycin is not effective at all against influenza or anything else except bacterial infections. (Influenza Drugs)

[73] Sandman PM, Lanard J., The Dilemma of Personal Tamiflu Stockpiling 10Jan2006

[74] Triage is a complex topic. I have expanded upon it considerably in an Original Article available on the BFM website entitled *Patient Prognosis and Triage During Pandemic Influenza.*

[75] The SOAP medical note format is part of the Problem Oriented Medical Record method developed by Dr. Lawrence Weed, MD. It is a useful way to record medical information on patients.

[76] Temperature can be measured in degrees F or C which ever is most familiar to you. In this manual, I use degrees in F.

[77] The pulse is usually regular, like a tom-tom drum. The beats are equally spaced and occur regularly. If you tap your toe to the pulse, a regular pulse is one that occurs predictably one beat after another. A regular pulse is normal. An irregular pulse is not. Having an occasional extra beat or drop beat is OK. A very fast irregular pulse can be a problem. This gets too complicated for me to give you specific advice except to say that a regular fast pulse in the context of flu suggests dehydration is present.

[78] Normal respiratory rates are in the range of 12 to 16 breaths per minute. Fever and dehydration are associated with faster

respiratory rates. Acidosis from massive infection is also a cause of high respiratory rates. When patients are near death, the respiratory rate slows down and becomes more and more shallow.

[79] Normal BP is 120/80 or so but there is a wide range of normal from a low of 90/60 for teens and girls to 140/90 for some adults. Pressures below 90/60 are usually abnormal and in the context of flu due to dehydration. These low BPs are often associated with a high pulse. Try to keep the patient's BP above 100 on the top and 60 on the bottom if possible.

[80] Fluid intake and output is best measured in milliliters (ml). Most kitchen measuring cups are graduated in both ml and ounces/cups.

[81] Fever, cough and shortness of breath are the three most common symptoms of Bird Flu in patients' admitted to the hospital with the disease in Southeast Asia from 2003 through July 2005. Adapted from: Avian Influenza A (H5NI) Infection in Humans. N Engl J Med 2005; 353:1374-1385 (Medical References)

[82] For the purposes of this book, ibuprofen means aspirin, Advil, Aleve, ibuprofen, or Nuprin since they are all alike. Acetaminophen (Tylenol) is not an aspirin.

[83] Dextromethorphan HBr is an antitussive (cough suppressant) that inhibits the cough reflex. It acts primarily by depressing the cough center in the brain to reduce the frequency of the intensity of cough. Prolonged use or high doses can cause confusions or hallucinations. DM is not very strong so if needed, switch to the opioid analgesic cough medicine. In the appendix you will find a recipe for home made cough syrup made from the ingredients found in the Flu Treatment Kit.

[84] Adapted from a chart found on Johnson and Johnson's Tylenol web site

[85] Tonghui MA, Verkman, AS., Aquaporin water channels in

gastrointestinal physiology. The Journal of Physiology, 1999; 517:2, pp. 317-326

[86] Sandle GI., Salt And Water Absorption In The Human Colon: A Modern Appraisal. Gut 1998;43;294-299

[87] *Survival and Austere Medicine: An introduction.* Written and edited by the Remote, Austere, Wilderness and Third World Medicine Discussion Board Moderators. April 2005 (Advanced Home Treatment)

[88] Bulter D., Wartime tactic doubles power of scarce bird-flu drug. Nature Vol:438, 3November2005

[89] Physicians as far back as ancient times practiced Uroscopy, the ancient art of urine inspection. This medical discipline was associated with the ancient school that believed that an imbalance in the humors or fluids in the body were the root cause of disease. The uroscopist collected urine in a special flask used to study its color, turbidity, and precipitates. The smell and taste were also used by the Uroscopist to judge the qualities of the urine. Specific qualities of interest were sweetness, bitterness, or saltiness. These early physicians used the character of the patient's urine to diagnosis illness and to establish their condition. In Medieval Europe, uroscopists were considered the leading practitioners of the healing arts and the flask they used in their art became the sign of the physician until its replacement with the stethoscope in the 17th century. The art of venerable practitioners of medical uroscopy was handed down to the modern day nephrologist and urologist.

[90] Azithromycin Product Circular (Influenza Drugs)

[91] This document is the property of the American Psychological Association and can be downloaded from the BFM website from the Home Influenza Treatment section.

[92] This topic is covered in greater detail on the BFM.com website as an Original Article entitled *Home Gardening During the Pandemic*

[93] Ragnar B., *The Survival Retreat*. 1983, Paladin Press, Boulder, CO (Books)

[94] Published in the British Medical Journal, December 22, 1979

[95] Stones A., Mass graves planned if bird flu pandemic reaches Britain. Daily Telegraph 2Apr2006

[96] From the FEMA Web site: *"How to ccorrectly boil or disinfect water. Hold water at a rolling boil for 1 minute to kill bacteria. If you can't boil water, add 1/8 teaspoon (~0.75 mL) of newly purchased, unscented liquid household bleach per gallon of water. Stir the water well, and let it stand for 30 minutes before you use it. You can use water-purifying tablets instead of boiling water or using bleach. For infants, use only pre-prepared canned baby formula. Do not use powdered formulas prepared with bleach treated water. Clean children's toys that have come in contact with contaminated water. Use a solution of 1 cup of bleach in 5 gallons of water to clean the toys. Let toys air dry after cleaning"*.

[97] On the BFM.com website I have placed a more in depth Original Article on this topic entitled *The Use of Household Bleach for Infection Control.*

[98] SODIS Solar Water Disinfection. EAWAG Aquatic Research http://www.sodis.ch/

[99] For a more thorough treatment of this topic, see *Stockpiling Food for the Influenza Pandemic* in the Original Article section of the BFM.com website.

[100] Stewart W., *How to Prepare for a Pandemic*. BookSurge, NY 2006 (Books)

182237

Made in the USA